Quick Start for Correctional Nurses

Medication Management in the Correctional Setting

Other books by Lorry Schoenly

Quick Start for Correctional Nurses:
Is Correctional Nursing for You?

The Wizard of Oz Guide
to Correctional Nursing

Correctional Health Care
Patient Safety Handbook

The Correctional Nurse Manifesto

Essentials of Correctional Nursing

Quick Start for Correctional Nurses

Medication Management in the Correctional Setting

Catherine M. Knox, MN, RN, CCHP-RN
Correctional Health Care Consultant

Gayle F. Burrow, MPH, BSN, CCHP-RN
Correctional Health Care Consultant

Series Editor
Lorry Schoenly, PhD, RN, CCHP-RN
Correctional Health Care Consultant

Enchanted Mountain Press

Quick Start for Correctional Nurses
Medication Management in the Correctional Setting

Copyright © 2016 Lorry Schoenly

CorrectionalNurse.Net

Published in the United States by Enchanted Mountain Press

ISBN: 978-1-9460410-0-5

Contents

Introduction to the Quick Start for Correctional Nurses Series

Welcome to the *Quick Start for Correctional Nurses Series* of brief books intended to jumpstart your correctional nursing practice. Each book in the series takes only an hour or two to read and is packed with essential and practical information on a specific topic important to correctional nurses. Some books cover nursing processes like sick call and medication administration while others deal with specific patient populations like female inmates or juveniles. Still others explore issues of concern to correctional nurses such as self-care needs and dealing with inmates.

Besides being packed with information, the Quick Start Series includes additional links and resources found on a special page of the CorrectionalNurse.Net blog. Access an expanding list of documents and links at correctionalnurse.net/quickstart.

Whether you are just discovering the world of correctional nursing, have started your first position in a jail or prison, or been in the field a while, the *Quick Start for Correctional Nurses Series* has something for you.

Introduction to Medication Management in the Correctional Setting

In the free world, individuals choose when and where to have their prescriptions filled. They also take their medication when and where they choose. In correctional settings, inmates must rely on nurses to ensure prompt and timely treatment with prescribed medication. In these settings, nurses are responsible for obtaining the medication from the pharmacy and then delivering it to the patient. The same is true of refills and renewals: Nurses have a pivotal role in ensuring that treatment is initiated promptly and that there is no discontinuity in prescribed medication. Correctional nurses must negotiate with all aspects of the system (custody staff, the court, providers, and pharmacy) to remove barriers that prevent prompt and timely treatment.

This Quick Start Guide provides nurses with the knowledge, tools, and resources to excel in managing medications while caring for patients in the correctional setting. Each chapter covers one aspect of medication management and includes questions that you can use to apply the information to your own setting. At the end of the book, we have provided links to additional information, tools, and resources that correspond to each chapter. The first of these tools, *A Simple Guide to Find Out How Medications Are Managed at Your Facility*, was designed to supplement your orientation and on-the-job training.

1 An Overview of Medication Management in Correctional Settings

It is your first day on the job, and another nurse escorts you to greet the Warden and meet with the Security Commander. Leaving the health care area, you must make your way through the line of inmates. It looks like a scene right out of the Jungle Book or Star Wars, with inmates in all manner of dress just standing around making the time of day with each other, but watchful at all times. As you make your way by, you hear catcalls and greetings to your colleague to ask if you are the new nurse. Your escort greets the inmates generally, but ignores the taunts and catcalls, walking briskly along the path to the Warden's office. As you leave the scene, you ask your colleague, "What are they all waiting for?" She answers, "Their meds." You think to yourself, "Wow, this is nothing like the way medications were administered at the hospital I just came from". Nurses who are new to the correctional setting are often unprepared for the scope and breadth of their role and responsibilities for managing medication delivery.

Principles of Medication Administration or Delivery

While correctional nursing is considered a specialty because it is different from other areas of nursing practice, the principles of nursing care are the same. It is only the setting (correctional facilities) and population (inmates) that define the differences. Correctional nurses must be skilled at adapting their practice to the setting and population, while retaining the principles that guide practice decisions. So, with regard to medication administration, the following principles apply:

- Medication is administered or provided to the patient consistent with a valid order that is specific to the patient and their condition.

- Treatment that is ordered must be provided. Delays in treatment should be minimized and cannot put the patient at risk of harm or injury.

- The patient provides informed consent before receiving medication and retains the right to refuse to take the medication.

- Medication administration should not conflict or interfere with inmate participation in meals, sleep, visiting, recreation, and work or program assignments. To prevent these conflicts, the time, methods, and location for medication delivery are a joint decision of the facility administrator and the health authority.

- The "rights" of medication administration are followed to ensure patient safety. These include at least the right patient, right medication, right dose, right route, and right time. More recently, these "rights" have been expanded to include right documentation, right reason, and right response.

- Medication practices (ordering, receipt, storage, and accountability) are consistent with state and federal laws, as well as facility procedures.

- Correctional nurses practice within the scope established in the state nurse practice act.

There is no "one way" to manage medications but, instead, many ways that nurses ensure that patients receive necessary treatment safely and securely in the correctional setting. Using these principles, you will be able to find workable solutions to resolve any issues that your patient or the setting present.

How Medications Are Delivered in the Correctional Setting

The American Nurses Association (ANA) notes that medication management is a primary responsibility of nurses working in correctional settings. A report from the Bureau of Justice Statistics, summarized in the table below, provides a glimpse of how many inmates are likely to be treated with prescription medication.

Table 1.1. Percentage of inmates who report taking prescription medication	Prisons	Jails
Inmates with chronic medical conditions	66%	40%
Inmates with mental illness	27%	15%

In addition to treating chronic medical problems and psychiatric disorders, medications are also prescribed for inmates who have acute conditions such as urinary tract infection, as well as to provide symptom relief for minor illnesses and discomfort such as headache, constipation or seasonal allergies. Added together, nurses may be responsible for ensuring that as much as 80% of the population at a correctional facility receives the correct medication and dose, at the right time and by the right route.

Nurse-administered Medication

The majority of medications in correctional facilities are administered by nursing staff to each patient, dose by dose. Nurses will most likely administer all medications in the infirmary or inpatient treatment units because the patient's condition or treatment needs closer monitoring. This procedure is very much like administering medications in health care settings in the community. Nurses also administer all medications in high custody areas (e.g. segregation, special management units etc.), not necessarily because of the patient's condition but because of the restricted movement of inmates in these units and a greater potential for misuse. In the general inmate population, nurse-administrated medication takes place when the patient's treatment needs close monitoring, the patient is incapable of taking it themselves, or when the drug has potential for misuse in the correctional setting.

Centralized vs Decentralized Delivery

Medication administration may take place in a centralized location such as the clinic, or it may be decentralized and take place in the housing unit. Within inpatient treatment units (mental health units, infirmary, and step-down programs), medication administration commonly takes place in the unit. In segregation or high-security areas, medication delivery will be decentralized and administered cell-side or in the pod.

Centralized medication delivery often takes place in a locked medication room in the health care area. The room usually has a locked Dutch door or window through which medication is passed to the patient. Medications for patients may be in drawers, cupboards, or carts behind this locked door. Inmates are called to medication line and wait until it is their turn to receive medication from the nurse at the pill window or door. Many nurses prefer centralized medication administration because of the backup and support provided by others in the health care area. Also, less time is spent traveling from one location to another with the medications and medication administration records (MARS). If something needs to be corrected, such as a medication that is not properly labeled, it can be taken care of at that moment rather than having to wait to get back to the clinic. Centralized medication delivery is, however, challenging for correctional facilities to manage movement to and from the medication window or cart, and it requires correctional staff to monitor the inmates waiting in line. Long medication lines impact other activities like meals, recreation, or visiting, and can become a hazard in the event of a security breach.

Decentralized medication administration involves taking the medication and the MAR to the patient, usually in a locked medication cart on wheels. The cart may be placed in the entry or by the officer's station in a housing unit. Patients come up to the cart one by one, and the nurse administers medication to each patient according to the MAR. Alternatively, the nurse may be expected to take the cart to the cell and administer medication to the inmate at the cell. Nurses may use back packs or bags, rather than a cart, to transport medications and MARs to the units for administration.

Self-administered Medication

Most people in the community take medication on their own. After a medication has been prescribed, the patient is expected to pick it up at a pharmacy or receive it in the mail. The patient then takes the medication on their own as instructed. Additional medication is obtained periodically until the prescription must be renewed. The patient then contacts their provider for a renewal. Most correctional facilities allow inmates to do the same because it is good preparation for release, is less staff-intensive, and does not interrupt other daily activities that take place in the institution. Correctional nurses provide patients with instructions about the medication, deliver the supply to the patient, check periodically to see of the patient is taking the medication as instructed, provides refills, and obtains renewal orders as necessary. Usually nurses deliver medication for self-administration at a time other than when administering medication.

Over-the-counter Medications

Some facilities allow inmates to obtain over-the-counter medications without having a prescription or seeing a health care provider first. In many cases, inmates are able to purchase items like aspirin, antacid, throat lozenges, vitamins, and skin products in the canteen or from the commissary. Sometimes these items are provided by the health services program upon request. Providing access to over-the-counter medications allows inmates to treat minor conditions in the same way they would if they were at home. Nurses may be involved in helping inmates learn about how to care for minor problems, such as dry skin or athlete's foot, themselves and may be expected to provide over-the-counter medications to inmates as necessary.

The Challenges of Medication Management

Managing patient medications in the correctional setting is one of the areas that distinguishes the specialty of correctional nursing from nursing more generally. The following challenges in medication management define correctional nursing practice.

Professional Isolation

Health care delivery in correctional facilities is often a very small part of the overall operation. In many cases, nurses are expected to deliver services independently and without advice or guidance from other health care providers. Dispensing, drug packaging, storage, inventory, and disposal of medications are all subjects governed by federal and state pharmacy laws and regulations. Correctional nurses need a strong working knowledge of all these requirements, in addition to general nursing requirements, to ensure compliance when responsible for medications in the correctional setting. Very often, a pharmacist is not on site and it falls to nursing staff to establish practices and find the resources to ensure compliance with pharmacy laws and regulations concerning dispensing, packaging, storage, inventory, and disposal of medication.

Expanded Role

Unless a correctional facility is large and has a number of specialized programs, the health care program is likely to be staffed without the support services nurses work with in other health care settings such as pharmacy technicians, IV teams, respiratory therapists, inventory clerks, and so forth. Nurses order medications from the pharmacy, arrange for refills and renewals, check for outdated drugs, receive, inventory and store medications, and arrange for medication to be returned or properly destroyed. Nurses are responsible to ensure that patients receive medication as ordered, this includes monitoring patient adherence and solving problems with medication availability.

Security and Safety Concerns

Maintaining security is a primary focus of correctional facilities. The most obvious example of a unique responsibility for correctional nurses is counting needles and syringes and accounting for each use. Correctional facilities are busy places with activities that compete with health care delivery and nurses must be vigilant to ensure that inmates receive medications when they are due. Correctional facilities are often crowded, with little privacy, so nurses also must be careful to protect patient confidentiality when administering medication. Nurses need to collaborate with security on an ongoing basis to ensure that access to patients who need medication and their privacy is maintained.

The safety of inmates, staff, and the general community is the other primary focus of correctional facilities. A significant aspect of medication delivery is managing inmate behavior. Nurses need to engage the cooperation and assistance of custody staff so that medication administration is conducted in a safe and efficient manner. Other patient safety concerns include infection control and preventing adverse drug effects.

Greater Volume and Scope

The volume of medication administered by a nurse in the correctional setting exceeds that in any other setting. Nurses are expected to administer many different medications that correspond to the range of diseases present in the population and to keep current with knowledge of new medications. Nurses may administer medication to patients in restraints, seclusion, or housed in a high security setting for disciplinary or protective reasons. Nurses sometimes administer medication involuntarily to patients with mental illness. In some correctional facilities, nurses may be expected to use PICC lines or other specialized equipment or procedures to administer medication.

Timeliness

Medication delivery and administration must take place in coordination with all of the other activities that compete for the time and availability of inmates. The nature of the correctional environment requires strict adherence to schedules, and this is beyond the immediate control of the nurse. Competition from other activities may impact the timeliness of medication administration and can affect the therapeutic effectiveness of the drug if given too close or far apart. Inmates who go to work or court before nursing staff are on duty may miss important doses unless the nurse makes arrangements for the medication to be kept on their person or taken to them when due.

See correctionalnurse.net/quickstart for links to several blog posts that elaborate on topics covered in this chapter.

Application Questions

Answers to the following questions will provide important information about your facility's approach to medication management.

1. What percentage of the population of inmates at your facility are prescribed medication?

   a. What percentage are taking medication for chronic disease?

   b. What percentage are taking medication for mental illness?

2. Is medication administration centralized or decentralized at your facility?

   a. How are medications administered to inmates in segregation?

3. Are inmates allowed to self-administer medications at your facility?

4. How do inmates obtain over-the-counter medication at your facility?

5. What is in your job description about medication management?

Case Example

The Facility Commander asks you for some ideas about how to reduce the time medication lines take at the minimum custody work camp where you work. Until now all medications have been administered by the nursing staff. Medication lines are impacting the times that crews report for their work assignments. What is the best idea you would suggest to the Commander and why?

2 Medication Management Guidelines, Terminology, and Information

Resources

As you get to know how medications are managed at your facility, remember that these practices are based upon laws and other regulations concerning nursing practice and the operation of pharmacies. Becoming proficient in medication services includes using the correct terminology to prevent communication mishaps and knowing how to access information resources. There is a lot to know, so don't expect to keep it all in your head. Knowing where to find information will help when you encounter unfamiliar situations.

Guidelines

Guidelines for medication management are established by the nursing profession, the individual state, and the federal government in laws defining professional practice acts and regulation of pharmacy services and in the standards for accreditation by professional organizations. Guidelines serve as the foundation for medication management procedures in place at your facility. Guidelines are the standard against which individual performance – as well as the program more generally – is measured. Correctional staff, including Wardens, are not necessarily knowledgeable about these and may request something that is not permitted. Knowing the guidelines and your facility procedures will help you avoid practices that are not permitted by law or regulation.

Nursing Standards

The ANA publishes a guide that describes the scope of practice and sets professional standards for correctional nurses. With regard to medication management, the roles and responsibilities of a correctional nurse are as follows:

1. Nurses must be knowledgeable of medications administered, including dosages, side effects, contraindications, and food and drug allergies.

2. Practices with regard to medication management in the correctional setting meet the same standards as in the community. To do so, nurses must be knowledgeable about state practice acts.

3. Nurses must ensure that patients know the names of all medications they are taking, the correct dosage, and potential side effects.

4. If patients are expected to take medications without supervision, the nurse evaluates the patient's competence to self-manage and takes steps to protect those who are not competent to do so.

5. Nurses work with custody staff so that patients receive medication in a timely and safe manner.

State Law, Rule, and Regulation

State law serves as the basis for nearly all of the practices and procedures involved in medication management. Most nurses are familiar with the nurse practice act in their state. If not, this is the place to start, by reviewing it for definitions and references to medication. The nurse practice act is particularly helpful in defining the training and supervision requirements of non-licensed personnel such as nursing assistants, emergency medical technicians (EMTs), and correctional officers, if they are expected to administer medication at the correctional facility.

In addition to medication administration, correctional nurses are often responsible for obtaining, storing, and accounting for the medications used to treat patients held in correctional facilities. This is because a pharmacist is usually not onsite. The pharmacy practice act is an excellent resource to find out how to manage medication at the facility. In addition to state pharmacy requirements, there are federal regulations that stipulate requirements about ordering, inventory control, and disposal of drugs. Even if there is a pharmacist at the facility, it is very important for each correctional nurse to be familiar with these regulations to better appreciate and understand why the pharmacist makes certain recommendations for drug storage, packaging of medications, and accountability. In addition to the facility's consulting pharmacist, the pharmacy board in your state is an excellent resource for information about state requirements and can help identify federal requirements that pertain to your facility.

The medical practice act is another important resource to review. It provides information about how a physician's order for medication is lawfully implemented. The medical practice act also has information about the work of medical assistants and EMTs, as well as their training and supervision, if these personnel are involved in medication management.

This is not interesting reading, but it does provide valuable information that nurses can use in sorting out the scope and limits of practice for each of the various personnel involved in medication management. It also provides definitions and terminology used to accurately communicate with the pharmacy and providers about implementation of orders. Finally, it provides nurses a basis to knowledgeably resist inappropriate requests from custody and other personnel, not familiar with health care laws, to perform tasks that are inconsistent with state law.

Case Example

Lynda is a nurse at a 1,600-bed adult male correctional facility. She is administering medications to inmates in segregation. One inmate who is objecting to being in segregation has been shouting obscenities at the officers for three days now. In addition, he has flooded his cell several times. The Unit Sergeant calls Lynda to his office and asks her to give the inmate something to calm him down. Lynda tells the Sergeant that there are no medication orders for the inmate. The Sergeant responds that he is ordering her to give the inmate a sedative. What should Lynda do?

Accreditation Standards

The National Commission on Correctional Health Care (NCCHC) and the American Correctional Association (ACA) are organizations that accredit correctional facilities. Even if accreditation is not sought, the standards are used by most correctional facilities in developing policy and practices. Both organizations have standards related to medication management, which are summarized in Table 2.1. This list is a handy description of all the moving parts and pieces of medication management in correctional facilities. Nurses are involved in all of these components. Use this list to review how medication is managed at your facility and identify areas that may need further attention.

Table 2.1: Standards for Medication Management in Correctional Facilities

	NCCHC	ACA
Applicable standards	C-05, D-01, D-02	4-4378, 4-4379
1.	Facility operates in compliance with state and federal laws regarding medications.	Similar
2.	There is a formulary and method to obtain non-formulary medication.	Similar
3.	Policy and procedures address how to procure, receive and account, dispense, distribute, store, administer, and dispose medication.	Similar
4.	Medications are under control of appropriate staff and accounted for.	Secure storage and perpetual inventory of controlled substances, syringes, and needles.
5.	Medication is only prescribed as clinically indicated after provider evaluation.	Similar
6.	Providers are notified of medication needing renewal prior to prescription expiration.	Similar
7.	Staff are properly trained to administer or distribute medication.	Similar
8.	Inmates do not prepare, dispense, or administer medications. Self-carry medication programs are allowed.	ACA does not address
9.	Outdated, discontinued, or recalled medications are not present at the facility.	ACA does not address
10.	If there is no onsite pharmacist, a consulting pharmacist is available for advice and makes inspections of the facility's medication program at least quarterly.	ACA does not address

Medication Management Terminology

The correct use of terminology enables nurses to communicate accurately and prevents misunderstanding with other nurses, providers, and pharmacy staff. The terminology used to describe who does what in the medication delivery system is subtle and often misused. In correctional settings, the most commonly misused medication terms are *dispense* and *administer*.

Dispense

This is the correct word to describe when more than one dose of medication is removed from a stock bottle or container, then labeled and packaged for a patient according to a written prescription (the sig). Only pharmacists and prescribers (physicians, advanced practice nurses, physician's assistants) can dispense medication. Important steps in this process are to verify that the order is safe (right drug for the problem, correct dosage, and route) and to review other medications the patient may be taking to ensure that the new medication does not cause an adverse interaction.

Administer

This is the correct term to describe when one dose of prescribed medication is given to a patient. Nurses (RN and LPN or LVN) are the primary professionals recognized by state law, who may administer medication. Medication administration involves not only correctly carrying out the order but assessment of the patient's response as well. Most states allow nurses to delegate the administration of medication to unlicensed personnel if they have been trained and are supervised.

Distribute or Deliver

Other types of personnel such as clerical staff, medical technicians, paramedics, and correctional officers may be lawfully involved in medication delivery in correctional facilities, specifically keep-on-person or over-the counter medications. The proper term for this is distribution or delivery of medication, not administration, because these personnel are not qualified to determine that the medication is being given as prescribed or to evaluate the medication's effect.

Nurses may be responsible for *procurement* and *accountability* of medication at the facility, especially if no pharmacy staff are onsite. This is not a role nurses have in traditional health care settings but is common in corrections.

Procurement

Ordering and receiving medication is referred to as procurement. An adequate number and variety of medications must be available at any time to treat inmate patients in a timely manner. To accomplish this, a correctional facility typically has an arrangement with a wholesale drug supplier or pharmacy to dispense and deliver patient-specific medications that are prescribed. In addition, a correctional facility will also procure stock supplies of medication to use in an emergency or to start treatment immediately.

Accountability

Medication accountability refers to the system used to track, document, and account for all medication – from the time it is received at the facility until it is administered or delivered to the patient, returned, or destroyed. Both state law and the accreditation standards require medication accountability in correctional facilities.

Terms to Describe How and Where Patients Receive Medication

There are a handful of terms used in correctional settings to describe how inmates receive medication. When inmates receive medication administered directly by a nurse, this is referred to as *directly observed therapy (DOT), watch-take, or nurse-administered meds.* Inmates may receive medication at *pill call or pill line* usually through a secure opening called a *pill window.* Alternatively, medication may be delivered to the patient in their cell or *cell-side,* through an opening in the door or come to a *pill cart* stationed in the housing unit. Sometimes the slang words used to describe an activity or place within a correctional facility are unprofessional or demeaning. For example, referring to the opening in the cell door as the "hash hole" is inconsistent with its use to deliver medication. Inmates may also receive a supply of medication to take on their own; terms used to describe this include *self-carry, keep on person (KOP), self-administered medication, or on- person medication (OPM).*

Formulary

As listed in Table 2.1, standards for correctional facilities require a *formulary,* which is a list of the medications that providers can order. If a particular medication is not on the formulary, there must be a way to request it for a particular patient if needed; this is called a "non-formulary" request. These requests are submitted to a senior physician or other designee such as the pharmacy manager, then reviewed and approved or denied. Correctional nurses are often involved in helping to fill out and track responses to "non-formulary" requests so the patient receives the medication in a timely manner. Having a record of non-formulary requests and a hard copy of each request can help reduce possible delays or interruptions in treatment. By knowing what is on the formulary, nurses can help providers by suggesting medications to avoid unnecessarily non-formulary requests.

Terms to Describe How Medication Is Packaged

Bulk stock is a supply of various medications from which a nurse takes out one dose for a particular patient. Bulk stock is maintained for use in an emergency and to administer initial doses of medication that cannot wait until the patient's prescription is delivered by the pharmacy.

For safety reasons, most state pharmacy laws now prohibit medication administration systems that rely solely on bulk stock and require instead *patient-specific packaging* that is in *unit dose*. Patient-specific packaging is a medication that has been prepared and dispensed by a pharmacist in a container or package that is labeled with the patient's name, start and stop date, the medication dose, route and frequency, and prescriber and pharmacy names.

Some medication is packaged in *unit dose* but is not patient-specific; examples are packets of two aspirin tablets or an inhaler, which are administered in the same manner as bulk stock. Usually several types of packaging are used in correctional facilities.

Information Resources

The types of health problems presented by our patients during incarceration is very broad, so it is necessary for correctional nurses to maintain knowledge about the full range of drugs likely to be prescribed. It is impossible to memorize all this information; having up-to-date references readily available is a must. The pharmacy that fills prescriptions for your facility may have a designated staff or resource line to answer drug information requests. You may find a similar resource at a nearby school of pharmacy or community hospital. Drug information today can also be accessed quickly in electronic format and is a very reliable reference for busy correctional nurses. See Table 2.2 for a list of recommended references that are available at no cost. Web addresses for each of these are also on correctionalnurse.net/quickstart.

Table 2.2. Resources for Medication Management
Drug Information Portal by the National Library of Medicine includes information on 56,000 drugs provided by journals, government agencies, and other noncommercial sources.
Drugs, Herbs and Supplements by the National Library of Medicine has drug information on intended uses, correct dosages, and drug interactions.
Pillbox is a database maintained by the National Library of Medicine that can be used to identify unlabeled pills.
Epocrates is a drug reference and includes a dose calculator, interaction checker, and pill identification material.
Medscape Mobile includes information on 8,000 drugs and supplements, a dose calculator, and robust drug interaction advice.

A final resource that should be available at every correctional facility is the telephone number for the poison control center. This national hotline number (800-222-1212) connects to the nearest poison control center. Most poison exposures can be treated locally with a poison control center because they are staffed 24 hours a day, seven days a week by health care professionals with special training. The individual correctional facility should also stock a supply of antidotes for various types of poison. See correctionalnurse.net/quickstart for a link to a consensus guideline published in the Annals of Emergency

Medicine, which recommended stocking 12 antidotes available for immediate use in treatment.

Availability of antidotes is a decision that should be made by the facility medical director in consultation with the supplying pharmacy based upon the likelihood of types of poisoning. For example, a correctional facility near a chemical plant or railroad will want to consider potential for chemical or gas disaster. Usually antidotes are stored with other emergency medications. Nurses should be familiar with each antidote stocked for use in medical emergency care. A web address to link to a list of common drugs and antidotes that nurses should know about can be found at correctionalnurse.net/quickstart.

The basis for your facility procedures can be found in the standards and guidelines. Using – and encouraging all coworkers to use – the correct terminology will prevent communication mishaps. Correctional nurses are expected to know a lot, often with little support, so having information resources is essential to practice safely in this environment. Be sure you know where to find the information when you need it.

Application Questions

Answers to the following questions will provide important information about your facility's approach to medication management.

1. Who administers medication at your facility?

2. How many different types of drug packaging are used?

3. Does your facility use a formulary? If so, what is the procedure to request a drug that is not on the formulary?

4. If the provider is going to prescribe an antidepressant and asks you which of these are on the formulary, how would you answer?

3 Reconciliation, Control, and Accountability for Medications

Inmate movement and change are inherent features of correctional settings, which require nurses to reconcile medication often to ensure continuity of patient care. Administering medications in a correctional setting also requires increased awareness of medication accountability and control. Concern for the security of medication begins on an inmate's entry into the system and continues throughout incarceration. Medication reconciliation practices, inventory controls, and pharmacy inspections are important processes to understand and maintain.

Medication Reconciliation

Medication reconciliation is a series of steps that are taken whenever there is a change in the patient's setting, condition, provider, or level of care. These steps verify what medications the patient is taking, determine what medications the patient's provider has prescribed, and resolve any discrepancies to ensure appropriate, timely continuation of treatment. Almost half of all medication errors in the general health care community occur because medication is not reconciled adequately when there is a handoff in responsibility for the patient's care, and 20% of these result in harm to the patient.

Transitions in the responsibility for an inmate's health care have the same risk. Inmates who have been taking medication prescribed by providers in the community will need to have those orders continued or modified by a provider when admitted to prison, jail, or other type of detention. Medication reconciliation also takes place when an inmate returns to the facility after receiving specialty care in the community, upon admission and discharge from infirmary or another type of inpatient care, and whenever their primary care provider changes. Medication reconciliation prevents mistakes in patient care.

Arriving with Medications

Offenders arriving at a facility from the community, especially jails and juvenile facilities, may have medications on their person; sometimes, family will bring in medications after learning their family member has been detained. It is best practice to verify that the medication received is the same as that on the label. Once verified, document the name of the medication, dose and frequency, date of filling, quantity remaining, physician, pharmacy, and prescription number. Verify the prescription with the pharmacy or community prescriber. Once this is done, notify the institution provider, who will determine if the medication should be started urgently so there is no lapse in treatment or if the patient should wait until seen for evaluation. There are several excellent sites for verification of drugs such as Drugs.com, Pillbox, and Epocrates.com. Links to each of these are found at correctionalnurse.net/quickstart.

Some institutions will allow the inmate to take medication brought in from home, if approved by the provider. If so, the amount received must be documented and acknowledged by the inmate. All doses administered must be accounted for by documentation on the MAR. When the inmate is released, all remaining doses (if any) are returned to the inmate in a properly labeled container. Some correctional facilities may place medications in the inmate's property, and others may give medications back to the family. Be familiar with your facility's policy about how patients' personal medications are handled.

Medications that Are Missing or Unavailable

Occasionally a patient will come to the med line or pill cart expecting to receive medication, and there is either no medication or MAR for the patient or the medication is not listed on the MAR. Asking the patient the following questions will narrow down where the medication may be located:

- Is this a new order? Have you ever taken this medication before?

- When was the last dose received? This indicates there is an active prescription and will help determine the urgency for resolution.

- When did you see the provider who ordered it? This is an important question to ask if the inmate hasn't had the medication yet. Maybe the prescription has not been dispensed yet, or perhaps it has arrived but hasn't been unpacked and put away.

- Have you been moved recently from another part of the facility? This indicates a need to check that medication and MAR were also transferred.

- When did you arrive at the facility? Or were you transferred from another facility? If so, check the transfer sheet. Medications and MAR may not have been transferred.

- Is it a prescription brought in from the community? The medication may be stored elsewhere.

- Have you gone by any other names? The medication may be filed alphabetically elsewhere.

Based upon the answers to these question, you will be able to advise the patient about the medication status or determine to resolve the issue by the next scheduled administration. Checking the patient's medical record and consulting with the pharmacy or provider may provide you with the information needed to respond to the patient's inquiry. If you are not able to resolve the problem promptly, be sure to assess the patient to determine if the provider should be contacted. Allowing patients to miss medication, even if somebody else is responsible, is equivalent to not providing treatment that is ordered. This could exacerbate their medical condition and can be a violation of their constitutional right to health care.

Offsite Care

Medication should also be reconciled whenever a patient returns to the facility from a hospitalization or specialty care. The clinical summary or recommendations by the offsite provider should accompany the patient; if not, the nurse should obtain this information right away. Recommendations from offsite specialists or hospital discharge instructions should be reviewed as soon as possible by the nurse and provider in order to continue the patient's care. When clinical recommendations from offsite care are missed or not followed up on, needed treatment is delayed and the patient's condition may deteriorate. There is a link to an article exploring this issue further at correctionalnurse.net/quickstart.

Chronic Care Patients

Chronic care patients are another group of inmates who require nursing attentiveness to medication reconciliation including:

- Evaluating whether the patient is actually taking the medication as ordered.

- Following up whenever the medication or the patient is not available and getting the missed scheduled doses to the patient promptly. Helping the patient to request refills and reorders in time may be necessary so doses are not missed. Account for the whereabouts of each no-show so that medication can be provided as scheduled.

- Often patients will refuse single doses or not pick up their KOP medications when they want to change or discontinue prescribed treatment. Each of these lapses should be discussed, the patient coached about the next steps to take, and the provider notified as well.

Accountability and Inventory Control

Regardless of the type of facility, accountability for each medication is required by state law. More importantly, since it is a correctional environment, control of all medication is paramount in preventing the endangerment of others that can result from medication diversion. Nearly 85% of incarcerated adults in the United States have a substance use disorder, and four out of five crimes committed by youth involve substance abuse. Prescription medication has a value in prison or jail that is greater than in the general community because access to illegal drugs is so greatly limited during incarceration. They are also used to trade or barter for other goods and services since exchange of money is not permitted between prisoners. Finally inmates may simply steal or trade for someone else's medication in an effort to alleviate insomnia, pain, anxiety, and boredom. The following paragraphs describe each of the processes involved in accounting for medications at correctional facilities.

Procuring and Receiving

The standard time for medication to arrive after an order has been submitted varies from one facility to another, depending upon the location of the pharmacy and its operating procedures. Waiting time may be as little as a few hours or as long as a week. Orders must be tracked and verified with each delivery. If any medications are missing, the pharmacy must be notified. If medication is on back order, the provider must be notified to decide if treatment orders should be modified. In addition, each medication should be checked for dispensing errors by reviewing the medication and label against the MAR or original provider order to ensure that it is the correct medication for the correct patient. Some correctional facilities have a pharmacy technician or clerical staff assigned to manage ordering and inventory control, but most facilities assign these responsibilities to nursing staff. Medications that are temperature-sensitive should be checked promptly and stored in the refrigerator or other appropriate temperature-controlled container.

Controlling Access

After medication has been dispensed by the pharmacy, it must be securely stored until administered or delivered to the patient. Usually this is in a designated room and only those nursing personnel with specific responsibility for medications have access. If medication carts are used, they are also stored in this room. The cupboards, drawers, or carts in which medication is stored are also locked when not in use. Keys are provided only to those personnel responsible for medication.

Medication storage areas must be organized, clean, and well-lit. All medications must be kept at proper temperatures, especially those requiring refrigeration. For more about the requirements for medication rooms, there is a link at correctionalnurse.net/quickstart.

Medication Administration Record (MAR)

The MAR is a record of each individual patient's medications and the last step in controlling medication inventory. The day and time medication is administered or delivered is documented on the MAR. Each time a new MAR is initiated or printed out, the nurse verifies that every medication listed is a current, active prescription by comparing the previous MAR against the new MAR *and* the order in the patient's health record.

Narcotics

Control of narcotics or controlled substances is of great concern to custody staff because of the risk these drugs present in a correctional facility. Controlled substances are stored under double lock but should not be so remote or difficult to access that delivery of patient care is impeded or inefficient.

Each controlled substance has a corresponding declining inventory or "proof of use" sheet. The date, time, quantity removed, name of the patient, and name of the person administering the dose is documented on the declining inventory log *and* on the MAR. At least once a shift, when nurses are on duty, one nurse counts the controlled substance medications and a second verifies that the remaining quantities match the documentation on the inventory sheet. If only one nurse is on duty, a member of the custody staff can assist with count verification.

Nurses who fail to account for controlled substances violate the state nurse practice act and the federal Controlled Substances Act; they may be at risk of criminal sanctions as well. Narcotic discrepancies result from a lack of documentation to account for each step in the administration of a controlled substance after removal of a controlled substance from the narcotic cabinet. Besides inaccurate documentation on the MAR, other discrepancies that indicate potential diversion, and are therefore best avoided, include:

- Signing out excessive doses;

- More sign-outs by a particular nurse;

- Lack of waste or excessive wasting;

- Documentation of medication administered for pain that does not correspond to the patient's rating of pain; and

- Lengthy periods of time between sign-out and administration to the patient.

Stock Medication

Stock medication is medication in bulk containers not labeled for use with a specific patient. Nurses obtain medication from stock containers to administer to patients according to the prescription. For patient safety reasons, most state pharmacy laws require medication to be packaged individually for each patient by a pharmacist or provider; this step creates a double check so that potential errors are identified and corrected before the medication reaches the patient. As a result, use of stock medication has diminished greatly in favor of patient-specific packaging.

However, some stock medication should always be kept on hand to initiate care immediately, when necessary. These occasions would include medical or psychiatric emergencies, infection and conditions when missing a dose is life-threatening (insulin, for example). Stock medications are also used in some situations because it is more cost-effective. Accountability for stock medications is maintained by logging the patient's name, date, time, quantity removed, and nurse's signature for each dose administered on a declining inventory log, similar to the log used to sign out controlled substances.

Inspections

A regular schedule is maintained at most facilities for inspection of the pharmacy, if one is onsite, as well as all the other areas where medication is stored. These inspections are usually conducted by the pharmacist who provides medication for the facility, but they may also be conducted by a pharmacist from the state board of pharmacy. A pharmacy inspection will look at practices in the following areas:

- Security of medications and medication areas;

- Cleanliness and order of work and storage areas;

- Temperature control of medication storage;

- Emergency medication availability and accountability;

- Inventory control;

- Sharps control;

- Controlled substance accountability; and

- References and reporting forms.

The pharmacy inspection may also include review of MARs to verify that doses are administered and documented correctly.

A copy of the inspection report is provided to the person responsible for health care at the correctional facility. Any areas found not in compliance with requirements for inventory, storage, and control of medications will be subject to corrective action.

Other inspections may be necessary to maintain licensure or certification of the pharmacy. Nurses should be aware of the licenses and certifications maintained by the site for pharmacy services, the requirements for each of these, and the dates for re-licensure or renewal. Finally, the Drug Enforcement Administration (DEA) may inspect the site to evaluate compliance with requirements for the facility's DEA license. A tool that lists the specific items covered in a typical pharmacy inspection, as well as a resource to prepare for a DEA inspection, can be found at correctionalnurse.net/quickstart.

Case Example

John has nearly finished his first month on the job at Merrimack Correctional Facility and feels like this new career choice is beginning to make sense. The delivery of medication from the pharmacy has just arrived, and along with the grocery bags of medication are two file boxes of MARs for the new month. John's co-worker groans and tells John that today they have to verify the old records to the new ones that just arrived. And as if that is not enough, the pharmacist has come along with the delivery and is going to conduct the quarterly inspection of the med room. The Health Services Administrator (HSA) sees the headlights in John's eyes and reassures him before he bolts: "Don't worry, help is on the way." Soon all available staff meet in the conference room to work on the MAR verification. The HSA and the pharmacist conduct the inspection together. Within an hour, the dust settles and staff are back to their other duties. The HSA stops by the medication room to see how John is doing and comments, "There are times when we have to come together to get a big job done, and this was one of those days." After a while, John is able to take these bumps in work flow in stride but knows that if he asks for help, it will be there for him. What has been your most challenging experience so far in medication management? What did you learn while addressing the challenge?

Application Questions

The following are some questions to use in getting to know how medications are reconciled and the procedures for medication control and accountability at your facility.

1. When do you obtain a list of medications the patient takes, and how do you verify the information provided by the patient?

2. How long does it take to fill a new order? What procedures are in place to obtain medication if it is needed before the pharmacy can fill the order?

3. What are all the inventory control practices in place at your facility? How are controlled substances accounted for?

4. How often is the temperature in the medication refrigerator checked? What steps do you take if the temperature in the refrigerator is too low?

4 Maintaining Security and Custody Support for Medication Administration

A collaborative relationship among nurses and correctional officers enhances the security of medications and timeliness of their administration or delivery. If correctional officers are unavailable or unwilling to help make sure inmates are available to receive medications, the patient will not receive ordered treatment. Not only may this put their health at risk, but it also violates the inmate's constitutional rights. If nurses are untrained, unwilling, or unable to control and account for medication and syringes, diversion occurs and significantly threatens the safety and security of all staff and inmates. Medication must be both kept secure and administered for the facility to accomplish its mission. Correctional nurses' actions must support both these requirements. The next few pages describe how this is done.

Security of Medication Storage

All health care facilities must provide for the security of medications until delivered or administered to the patient. This is even more important in correctional facilities where unsecured or unaccounted medication is considered contraband and a major security breach.

Pharmacy

If there is a pharmacy onsite, access is usually limited to staff who work in the pharmacy. Nurses, providers, and others may drop off prescriptions, pick up medications, or exchange information with pharmacy staff through a window or in an anteroom to the pharmacy. During hours when the pharmacist is not onsite, access will either be prohibited or extremely limited, with any entry documented and accounted for.

Medication Storage Areas

Nurses administer medication from a medication room or a medication cart (or bag). Medication rooms are locked when not occupied, and access by others is controlled and/or restricted. Medications stored in these rooms are kept in locked cabinets. If there is a "pill window," it is kept locked except when medications are being administered. Medication carts are stored in a medication room or other locked area when not in use. Medication carts are locked except when in use.

Controlled substances are stored in a separate cabinet or drawer that is locked except when medication is withdrawn or being stocked. Some facilities use automated dispensing cabinets to store medications, which is especially useful for narcotics, stat doses, or starter packs of medication. These machines require a unique sign-on, document all transactions, and create discrepancy alerts.

Only the nursing staff who are responsible for medication should have keys to the medication room and carts. Typically, access to the narcotic cabinet is limited to one nurse. Other nurses needing access to the narcotic cabinet obtain the key from the nurse who is responsible for it and return the key when finished.

Emergency Medications

Emergency medications are stored in a container (i.e. an emergency kit or "man down bag") that is ready to take when responding to the event. A double lock is accomplished by locking the door to the room or cabinet that emergency medications are stored in and then locking the box, pocket, or container in which the drugs are stored. The emergency medication and equipment should be checked during each shift in which health care staff on duty to verify that the locks are intact and the equipment is functional. This verification is documented on a log. Plastic numbered tags can be used to "lock" the container where the emergency drugs are stored. If used, the number on the tag is recorded on the log documenting that the emergency equipment has been checked. Usually one staff member each shift is responsible for emergency response; this person will verify that the locks are intact and document verification on the log.

Sometimes medications may also be stored in provider exam rooms so that, when necessary, treatment can be started immediately. An acceptable way to ensure security of these medications is to have the provider sign out a box of stock medications, take it to the exam room, and put it in a locked drawer. At the end of the clinic, the provider returns the box of stock medications (and an accompanying sheet that documents what medication was dispensed) to the pharmacy or medication room.

Security Precautions for Medications

Medication administration and delivery takes place several times each day. Whether it is done correctly and on time effects nearly everyone in a correctional facility. Here are the security precautions related to medication administration and delivery in correctional settings.

Nurse-administered Medications

The security advantage of nurse-administered medications is that nursing staff "control" all medications and there is less likelihood of misuse. Security staff have the responsibility to supervise medication administration to ensure that inmates get to the nurse promptly, maintain order among inmates waiting for medication, prevent the nurse and medication cart from being crowded, and assist with medication refusals. The following are standard security practices during medication administration:

- Nurses should use two-part identification to verify that the correct inmate is receiving the correct medication (i.e. name and identification number), even if the inmate is known to the officer or the nurse.

- Inmates should be observed swallowing medications to prevent hoarding. This includes checking the inmate's mouth and hands to prevent diversion.

- Inmates should be instructed about medication side effects and encouraged to report any possible side effects they experience.

- Together, nurses and officers should account for the reason why any inmate does not appear to take their medication (e.g., at court or a medical appointment, has a visitor, has been transferred, or has not been let out of the cell).

Self-administered Medications

Medications eligible for self-administration are limited to those with low potential for misuse. The facility administrator, warden, or superintendent (with input from health services) determines which medications may be self-administered based upon the type of population and experience controlling contraband. The security aspects of self-administered medication include the following principles:

- Clear instructions for inmates about their roles and responsibilities, including securing medication in their property and consequences of violation. See correctionalnurse.net/quickstart for a good example of inmate instructions.

- Documentation on the MAR that the inmate received their medications by having the inmate sign and date the receipt of medication with a notation of the quantity provided.

- Any medication for self-administration must be labeled with the inmate's name, identification number, date filled, medication, dosing directions, and quantity given.

- Custody staff should confiscate any medication not found in the correct inmate's property and notify health services.

- Nurses should randomly check on inmates who self-administer medication to ensure that they are taking it correctly, confirm the patient's understanding of the rules for self-administration, and make certain that they know how to obtain refills.

Over-the-counter Medications

Over-the-counter medication may be available for inmates to purchase in the canteen, and they may be available at the officer's desk or in the health care area. Many facilities make medications used to manage symptoms of headache, common cold, and indigestion available to inmates as needed because it reserves the time and resources of a sick call for those health care problems that require professional judgment to determine the course of treatment. The security features in place to prevent misuse of over-the-counter medications include the following principles.

- Limited types of medications available;

- Limited quantity that inmates can have at any one time; and

- Inspection of medication containers for potential harmful use such as making a weapon or hiding contraband.

Preventing Diversion of Medication

Diversion of medication has always been a concern of custody staff, but now that many more medications are available and considered part of medically necessary treatment, the risk and opportunity for diversion has increased. Diversion and misuse of prescription medication is as much a clinical problem as a custodial one. If patients are bullied or coerced into giving up needed medication, their condition may deteriorate. The provider may then prescribe higher doses or additional medications to treat a condition that appears unimproved when, in reality, the patient simply has not been treated effectively in the first place. And when an inmate takes someone else's medication, they are not monitored clinically and expose themselves to adverse reaction or other injury. Correctional nurses should be hyper-vigilant when administering medication with high diversion value. A link to a list of prescription medications that are commonly misused or abused by inmates can be found at correctionalnurse.net/quickstart. This resource also lists the purpose each drug is usually prescribed for and common reasons for its misuse. Please remember, though, that any prescription medication can be misused if there is a belief that the drug will produce some desired effect. Here are some ways to prevent diversion of medication in correctional facilities.

Vigilance for Risk of Diversion

The nurse should watch closely for behaviors indicating that a patient is "at risk" for drug diversion, document their findings in the inmate's health record, and inform the patient's prescribing provider. This information is more helpful to the treating provider when it is descriptive rather than judgmental. Indications that a patient may be "at risk" of diverting prescribed medication include:

- Requesting a particular drug by name before describing symptoms;

- Inconsistencies between objective data about the patient's condition and the description of symptoms;

- Refusal or non-adherence with other drugs prescribed for the condition;

- Claiming allergies or side effects to other possible drugs without being able to provide specific details;

- Not remembering or being able to pronounce drugs other than the preferred drug; and

- Threatening or other signs of excessive distress when the requested drug is not prescribed.

Nurses should also discuss with patients the potential for their victimization when taking medication, the adverse outcomes of prescription drug abuse, and steps to protect themselves. This discussion is most effective if it is specific to the patient, the drug, and their behavior.

Increased Multidisciplinary Communication

Communication between providers, nurses, and custody staff about prescription drug abuse and the importance of minimizing diversion will reinforce the roles of each in doing so. Correctional officers should be invited to provide information about behavior that suggests coercion by others or diversion. Random cell searches by correctional staff and periodic review of adherence by nursing staff are very helpful in identifying inmates who are diverting medication.

Case Example

You see an inmate at sick call today for a complaint of low back pain and a request for gabapentin. He is well-known to you because he comes to sick call frequently, usually about his back or some other musculoskeletal injury. Today his vital signs are normal, he has not had a recent injury, and he reports no other change in his condition. His gait is normal; when asked to bend over, reach, and so forth, you see no sign of stiffness or guarding. Other aspects of the physical exam are normal. The provider saw this patient last month and did an extensive work-up for low back pain, including prescribing exercises and a mild muscle relaxant. You ask the inmate to demonstrate one of the exercises, and he cannot remember how it is done. You look at his MAR for the month, and he seems to be taking the muscle relaxant as ordered. He says that the doctor at the last facility prescribed gabapentin for him, and it worked very well. You discuss the case with his provider and comment that he seems at risk for diversion. What data from your evaluation will you use to support your concern?

Formulary Controls

A common reaction to diversion is to ban prescription of a certain drug. The problem with this approach is that, once a particular drug is banned, another becomes the drug of choice for misuse. Secondly, there are appropriate clinical indications for each medication, and not allowing its use may amount to denial of medically necessary care. As an alternative to banning a particular drug, drugs with diversion value can be designated as non-formulary, which requires additional rationale and review before it can be issued. It is also possible to designate a certain location with greater supervision and control to house patients receiving drugs at high risk for diversion.

Form of Drug Preparation

Another option is to administer the drug in a way that limits the possibility of diversion. Choices include ordering the drug in a liquid, aerosol or injectable preparation or that the tablet be "crushed and floated." Challenges are that these methods are more expensive, very time-consuming to administer, and can alter the drug in a way that makes it unsafe. A policy to "crush and float" an entire class of drugs (i.e. psychotropics) is not advised. Nurses expose themselves to liability if they "crush and float" medications against manufacturer advice. See Chapter 5 for more strategies to protect yourself and your patients if crushing and floating medication is being considered.

Sharps Control and Narcotic Counts

Counting Sharps

A distinguishing feature of correctional nursing practice is accounting for needles, syringes, and other medical instruments. This is necessary because sharps can be used as weapons, for tattooing, and for injecting drugs, which are all dangerous and prohibited activities in a correctional facility. A missing sharp means that the whole facility may be locked down and searched until the item is found. No other work, not even delivery of health care, takes place until the missing sharp is accounted for.

Sometimes nurses balk at the requirement for counting or act as though it isn't as important as patient care. On the contrary: Failure to account for sharps is not only dangerous but also undermines the professional relationship with custody staff. One tip for easing the burden of sharps count is to reduce the inventory to only the amount and type that are needed for that day or week. This is referred to as active inventory. These sharps need to be signed out as they are used, and the remainder is counted every shift by the health care staff on duty. Additional inventory can be kept in another locked cabinet with restricted access and documentation of sign-out. The backup inventory needs to be counted only after the cabinet has been unlocked. Another is to have an inventory count sheet for each type of sharp. Keep these organized in a binder or folder that corresponds with how the count is conducted (for example, by drawer or shelf, or alphabetically).

Counting Narcotics

Virtually all nurses are accustomed to counting narcotics in health care settings. The same expectations apply in correctional settings, including:

- Sign-out of each dose from the narcotic storage cabinet, drawer, or other locked container is done just before the dose is due to be given.

- The sign-out record includes the nurse's signature, the patient's name with other patient identification, the time, date, and the quantity removed.

- The same nurse must administer the narcotic and document administration on the MAR.

- If the dose is not given, the MAR should reflect the reason.

- When unused medication can be returned to stock, the narcotic sheet reflects the date and time, the addition, the reason, and the signature of the nurse on duty.

- Two staff members must witness a wasted dose and document the wasted dose, date, and time with signatures on a destroyed narcotics log.

- The narcotic count should be verified and documented by two people at the start and end of each shift when health care personnel are on duty. If only one health care staff member is on duty, the other person verifying the count can be a member of the custody staff.

Reviewing practices periodically can be helpful in identifying and correcting potential gaps or poor practices that enable loss of medications.

Application Questions

The following questions can be used to review practices in maintaining medication security at your own facility.

1. How many locations are used to store medications at your facility? Are they under double lock when not in use?

2. Consider your own security practices – for example, do you lock the medication cart or cabinets when you leave the area, even just for "a moment"?

3. What are the security aspects of nurse-administered medication that your facility uses?

4. If you were the only nurse on duty at a correctional facility, how would you count controlled substances?

5. What do you do if you suspect an inmate of diverting their prescription medication?

5 Safety Considerations for Staff and Patients

There is much written in the health care literature about patient and staff safety in the general health care community. The same concerns apply in correctional nursing. In addition to the safety issues involved in health care delivery, the correctional environment has its own risks that demand additional nursing attention. The next few pages provide information about how to keep your patients and yourself safe when managing medications in correctional health care.

Staff Safety

Staff safety is achieved primarily by ensuring that other staff are in the area and are aware of the nurse's presence and activity, controlling inmate movement, minimizing distractions, and maintaining expectations for appropriate inmate attire and behavior. Nurses contribute to staff safety by maintaining a professional demeanor, monitoring the medication cart and keys, minimizing distractions, maintaining an awareness of the correctional officers' presence and activity, and responding to information provided by the officer.

Custody Escorts

When nurses administer medication in health care settings, they do so alone. By contrast, the cooperation and assistance of custody staff are essential when you administer medication to patients in correctional settings. This assistance is provided to protect your personal safety, to control access to medications, and to protect inmates from harm. An officer may actually accompany you as you go from unit to unit, or the officer in each unit may stand by as you administer medication. An officer may escort inmates to the medication cart or to the clinic, or an officer may stand outside the pill window watching inmates as they wait in line.

Staff involved in medication administration (nursing staff as well as correctional officers) should receive initial and periodic training about the facility's processes and security in delivering medication, according to the accreditation standards of the American Corrections Association (ACA) and the National Commission on Correctional Health Care (NCCHC). While custody staff have a different professional worldview from nurses, both perspectives are valuable; do not feel compelled to become a correctional officer to adapt to this setting, and don't expect them to adopt your values. Nurses who retain their nursing perspective and practice consistent with nursing standards while abiding by security requirements ultimately gain officers' respect.

The kinds of tasks that correctional officers may be assigned in support of medication administration include:

- Using an accurate roster of inmates who are scheduled to receive medication at a specific time.

- Providing the names and whereabouts of any inmates not on the unit at the time.

- Announcing that it is time for medications.

- Suspending other activities that interfere with medication administration.

- Lining inmates up and maintaining order during medication line.

- Preventing inmates from gathering around or crowding the nurse.

- Assisting with identification of each inmate.

- Observing each inmate swallow medication and dispose of the medication cup.

- Mustering inmates who do not appear for medications when called.

- Escorting inmates who refuse medication to the nurse for counseling and to sign the refusal. If the inmate refuses to sign the refusal, the nurse may document this on the refusal form, and the officer may witness and co-sign the nurse's notation.

A nurse can contribute to the working relationship with custody staff by acknowledging and expressing appreciation for the assistance they provide.

Personal Safety

Nurses can take these steps to protect their personal safety while administering medications:

- Be aware of inmate behavior as you administer medication. Usually you can spot someone beginning to escalate well before they are in front of you asking for meds. Also cue into the information that correctional officers have about the behavior of specific inmates under their supervision.

- Be vigilant about the medication cart and its placement. Keep heavy objects like the pill crusher out of sight when not in use. Lock the brakes so the cart can't be shoved. Don't let inmates crowd your work space, lean on the cart, or stand or walk behind you.

- Keep control of your keys. Don't carry unnecessary keys or other items.

- Dress in conservative attire appropriate for medication administration.

- Make sure that there is a member of the custody staff nearby and actively monitoring inmate behavior. You can't be both the cop and the nurse at the same time. It certainly is appropriate to correct or challenge inappropriate inmate behavior, but it is not your duty to manage safety/security and medication administration all at once.

Maintaining Order

What may seem routine for custody staff on a housing unit, in the hallway, or out in the yard can quickly become distractions, waste time, lead to misunderstanding, and increase the risk of error during medication administration. It is best to eliminate distraction by having the television turned down, the lights turned on, and other competing activity or movement suspended while medication is being administered. Nurses should adhere to schedules and communicate with correctional officers about their progress with medication administration. Correctional officers usually announce when it is time for medications after the nurse indicates that they are ready to proceed. If inmates aren't ready and don't come to get their medications promptly, medication delivery is prolonged and other activities are delayed, which inconveniences everyone and can cause a disturbance. A correctional officer should manage a steady flow of inmate traffic to the nurse or escort the nurse if going cell to cell is necessary.

Managing Behavior

Medication administration is also an opportunity for some inmates to act out. Common examples include sleeping in, showing up late, and refusals. When this behavior goes unchallenged, it defeats the purpose of treatment. The custody staff should muster those who should but do not appear for medication administration, even those who are refusing. Only you can accept a refusal directly from the patient; it cannot be based upon the officer's report. This is because the nurse needs to ascertain the reason for the refusal and determine if there are any immediate clinical concerns. Patients who sleep in or refuse medication repeatedly should be brought to the attention of the provider and their prescriptions reviewed to see if adherence can be improved.

More extreme examples of disorderly behavior include yelling, pervasive use of profanity, throwing body fluids, and masturbation. No nurse is expected to administer medications under threatening or abusive conditions. If this happens, inform the officer that you will return when the unit or behavior is under control, and immediately inform your supervisor. Sometimes this can be an ongoing problem on a particular unit or with a particular inmate. In these cases, nursing staff should be included in problem-solving or at least provided with information about what is being done to ensure their safety and to get medication delivered.

Patient Safety Issues Unique to Correctional Settings

Patient safety with regard to medication management is a priority in health care today, and that same concern extends to correctional health care. The correctional setting provides some unique challenges to both medication management and patient safety. Here are some key patient safety concepts as they apply in the correctional setting.

Order Verification

Verbal orders are more common in correctional health care because providers are not onsite as often compared to traditional health care settings. Verbal orders should be limited to urgent patient care and not a routine practice or convenience – misunderstandings regarding dose or medication name are just too common when orders are provided verbally.

Safety precautions when taking a verbal order include the following best practices:

- Write the order down exactly as you hear it.

- Repeat the order back to the prescriber, reading directly from the order as you have written it.

- Spell out the medication name and dosage (i.e. t-w-o milligrams).

- Have the prescriber affirm that the order, as you repeated it back, is correct.

- Have the prescriber co-sign the order the next time he/she is onsite.

Patient identification

Patient identification is an area where correctional nurses can become lax. The reasons for this are:

- The inmate may be very well-known to them.

- The nurse is pressured for time.

- Inmates won't provide their identification number or birthdate when asked.

- Independent identification (i.e. ID card, wrist band, or badge) is not easily accessible.

Inmates may purposely misrepresent themselves at med line, giving another patient's name and receive that patient's medication. It is less likely that they will know the other person's birthdate or identification number and thus the reason why two-part identification is so important. Use of photo identification is recommended, as it enhances the likelihood of identifying the right person in the case of an inmate who has gained knowledge of another person's identifiers. Another reason for the emphasis on patient identification is that some patient names are identical or very similar to others, and/or they may go by several names. When there are similar, identical, or common names, use name alert stickers and add aliases on the MAR to guarantee it is the right patient.

Infection Control

Concern for infection control should be paramount in your mind every minute you are in a correctional facility. When you think about the number of people who come through the facility, the surfaces they touch, what their hygiene may be, the quality of ventilation, water temperatures, and so forth, the possibilities for infection can be significant.

If a medication cart is used, it should be cleaned with an appropriate surface cleanser before each use. If medication is administered from a room, the ledge or counter used to prepare medication should be cleansed before use.

If water is provided, the container should have a disposable liner that is changed each time it is used. Because liners are used, the container only needs to be cleaned with a 10% bleach solution once a week. If liners are not used, the container needs to be cleaned before each use with an appropriate cleanser. Patients should not touch the water dispenser handle, so the nurse should pour and hand the cup to the patient. If patients bring their own water, their cups should not be placed on the medication cart or window ledge, and the nurse should not have contact with it.

The nurse should sanitize their hands before administering medication, after rolling the cart to a new location, and anytime an object not on the medication cart or work area is touched (e.g. door knob, gate, buzzer, etc.). Having an alcohol-based hand sanitizer on the medication cart or nearby in the medication room facilitates hand hygiene.

Privacy and Confidentiality

Medication administration in correctional facilities is usually conducted in a semi-public setting (e.g. day room, hallway, corridor, cell block), and patient confidentiality can be compromised as a result. Other inmates waiting for their medication are alert to what you are saying while administering medication to the patient at the front of the line or in the next cell. While it is important to converse with the patient about their medications, symptoms, and side effects, how and what you can say while administering medication will depend upon how much privacy there is. When auditory privacy cannot be assured, your conversation should be more general and you should follow up by arranging for the inmate to visit the clinic later.

Case Example

While administering medication, the housing unit officer was busy talking on the telephone. Inmates were talking to one another while waiting in line and beginning to act out, telling jokes and egging each other on. Soon one inmate jumped ahead of another and used that inmate's name and identification number. The nurse observed what happened and stopped preparing medication. What are some of the things the nurse would be thinking about doing in this situation?

Best Practices to Prevent Medication Errors

Nurses are at the "sharp end" of medical errors. What this means is that the nurse is the last point between the patient and the medication. Thus they can prevent harm to patients by discovering errors before the patient takes the medication. This could include a misunderstood order, a mistake in dispensing or labeling the medication, mistakes in filling, and mistakes in preparation. Being the last stop before the patient means that the safety practices of the nurse during medication preparation and delivery are critical for preventing harm to the patient.

Defining Medication Error

Medication error is not limited only to those occasions when a patient is harmed. Now the definition of a medication error is broader and includes any *preventable* event where medications *may* be *used inappropriately or cause harm* while the medication is in control of the health care professional or patient. Examples of errors where the patient was not harmed are when the wrong drug is put in the patient's cup but the patient's notices and tells you, or you discover that a medication has not been packaged correctly and call the pharmacy. Most medication errors occur not because nurses are malicious or incompetent but arise instead from poor practices, inadequate equipment, poor communication, incomplete procedures, and other systemic issues in the organization. These system failures can only be identified by examining errors and creating opportunity to develop solutions that prevent the error from happening again.

Implementing Medication Orders

An order for medication travels through many "hands" before it is administered to a patient. There are many opportunities for misunderstanding along this continuum, so it is important that the written order be complete, legible, and accurate. The main components of a medication order include:

- The patient's first and last name. If it is a common name, include the middle name as well;

- Case, record, or identification number unique to the patient;

- Date and time the order is written;

- Specific medication name;

- Medication strength or dosage;

- Directions for use, such as how many times and at what time of the day;

- Route to give the medication, such as by mouth, intramuscularly, or inhaled;

- Allergies documented or no known drug allergies (NKDA) noted;

- Special instructions for taking the medication, such as with a meal;

- Duration of the order, number of pills, or stop date; and

- Prescriber's legible signature and credentials.

A nurse should review orders soon after they are written and seek clarification if it is unclear, illegible, incomplete, or incorrect so that treatment is not delayed.

Transcribing Orders

Many correctional facilities have greatly simplified order implementation with computerized provider order entry and prescription labeling, electronic generation of the MAR, and electronic documentation of medication administered. If you are lucky enough to work in a facility with computerized provider order entry (CPOE), nursing staff will not have to transcribe new orders, except in the case of a treatment that cannot wait until the pharmacy delivers. In that case and for those who work in facilities without this kind of automated support, order transcription involves the following steps:

1. Usually new orders are routed to a specific nurse who transcribes it onto the MAR exactly as it is written by the provider. Transcription may be delegated to nursing assistants or clerical staff, but the nurse retains responsibility for review and follow-up that the transcription was done correctly.

2. After the order is written on the MAR, the nurse checks the MAR against the order and notes that it has been correctly transcribed by signing and dating the order itself. This communicates to the provider that ordered treatment has been initiated. If the task has been delegated, the nurse must verify that the transcription is correct by reviewing the orders and MAR and then initialing the order.

3. The order is then sent by the nurse (or delegate) in electronic form or by fax to the pharmacy to fill and dispense.

Because of the potential for transcription error, best practices include applying a sticker directly on the MAR that includes all of the information about the order or using a preprinted medication sheet, both of which can be supplied by the pharmacy. In a fully automated medication system, the electronic MAR will be updated at the time the medication is dispensed and only needs to be printed to document administration when the system is down.

Preventing Miscommunication

Even when we speak the same language, communication can be misunderstood. Errors in communication occur in oral and written communication about medications, and sometimes these result in adverse consequences for the patient. One example is QD (daily), often misunderstood as QID (four times daily) resulting in four times the intended daily dose. The opposite is also true, but the patient would receive a much lower dose than was intended therapeutically. Either error can have disastrous consequences.

The Joint Commission (TJC), the U.S. Food and Drug Administration (USFDA), and the Institute for Safe Medication Practices (ISMP) have each promoted practices that reduce errors in communicating about medications. Your facility should have a list of approved abbreviations and may also have a list of abbreviations to avoid using because they are prone to error. If not, see correctionalnurse.net/quickstart for a list of medication abbreviations that are frequently misunderstood.

Eight Rights of Medication Administration

We all learned in our nursing education about the five "rights" for medication administration. Over the last decade, three more rights have been added to increase the emphasis on patient safety and error reduction. These are listed in Table 5.1 along with the nursing practices that ensure the "right" is met. By following these practices, nurses can identify and prevent medication errors from harming the patient.

Table 5.1. Nursing Practices Consistent with the Eight Rights of Medication Administration

Right Patient: Check the name on the MAR, and use two patient identifiers; ask the patient to identify themselves, then check the name &/or picture on the ID wrist band or badge.

Right Medication: Check the order, select medication, compare to the order, check the MAR, then check the medication against the MAR before giving to the patient. If it is a new medication, check that the patient knows what it is for and whether any patient allergies contradict giving it.

Right Dose: Check the order or the MAR, and confirm the appropriateness of the dose. For medications with high-risk consequences from dosing errors, ask someone to double-check the calculation.

Right Route: Check the order and MAR, confirm that the route is the correct for that medication and dose, and confirm that the patient can receive it by the ordered route.

Right Time: Check the frequency the medication is to be given on the MAR, verify that the time is correct for this dose, and confirm when the last dose was given.

Right Documentation: Document administration AFTER giving the medication; document the route, time, and other specifics (such as site, if injectable), as well as lab values, pain scale, or other data as appropriate.

Right Reason: Confirm the rationale for the ordered medication: Why is it prescribed? Does the patient know why they are taking this medication? If they have been taking it for long, is its continued use justified?

Right Response: Has the drug had its desired effect? Does the patient verbalize improvement in symptoms? Does the patient think there is a need for an adjustment in the medication? Document your monitoring of the patient for intended and unintended effects.

(Adapted from Bonsall, 2011. 8 rights of medication administration.)

Patient Involvement

A last tip to prevent medication error is to involve your patient. The more informed patients are about the medications they are taking, the reasons why, what symptom improvement to expect, how to manage side effects, and when to seek help, the more effectively they can assist in monitoring their condition. An involved and informed patient can be another safety check to prevent medication error, but you have to give patients a way to communicate with you effectively, and they need to know what to expect.

Reporting Errors

Reporting and reviewing all errors, even those that did not harm the patient, provides information about how to prevent another occurrence that may cause harm to a patient in the future. Your facility should have an established process for reporting medication errors. Error reports should be reviewed to determine what steps can be taken to prevent error in the future. These reviews result in changes in how medication is ordered, dispensed, delivered, prepared, and administered at your facility. Having a workplace philosophy and culture that emphasizes the importance of finding errors in support of patient safety provides assurances that improvements will be made and staff supported in their work.

Risky Medication Administration Practices

For various reasons, every nurse has likely engaged in one or more of the risky practices discussed in this section. Every time these practices are used, the patient's safety is put at risk. We have an obligation to practice in ways that lessen patient risk. Sometimes nurses encounter longstanding facility practices that involve one or more of these practices. If so, we suggest ways to lessen risk with each type of practice, but nurses are encouraged to speak up about patient safety concerns and to seek alternative practices as soon as possible.

Tablet Splitting

Cutting a pill in half to give a smaller dose may seem like a cost-saving measure, but it can also cause patient harm because it affects the drug's potency or absorption. Tablet splitting also eats into valuable nursing time that could be spent instead seeing patients. You might review this resource if you are asked to split tablets and then consult with the pharmacist for guidance.

Crushing

Besides the time it takes to crush, some crushed medications also do not absorb correctly or cause damage or irritation to the stomach. The Institute for Safe Medication Practices (IMSP) has published a list of medications that should not be crushed. Here are some recommendations if crushing medications is being discussed or is expected:

- Attempt to find the drug in another form (liquid or injectable).

- Crushing should be written as part of the individual patient's order.

- Limit crushing to high-risk medications or high-risk patients.

- Check to make sure it is a medication that can be crushed.

- Use individual packets if it is a communal crushing device to eliminate the potential of mixing medications.

- Do not mix crushed medications together, and do not administer with food or juice to prevent harmful interactions.

Staging or Pre-pouring

The practice of putting medications up in cups or envelopes prior to administration is a very risky practice and should only take place in unavoidable situations. It sometimes done in segregation housing when the medication carts cannot go up a narrow flight of stairs and medications are delivered from cell to cell. A solution to this is to use a notebook binder, basket, or bag with just the medication for that tier and related MARs. Nurses sometimes prefer to pre-pour so that they spend less time in front of inmates, but this defeats the safety measures of patient-specific packaging and limits the opportunity to evaluate how patients are doing. If you find that you must pre-pour, there is a resource about the safety principles related to staging medications at correctionalnurse.net/quickstart.

An even more risky practice is to pre-pour for someone else or to administer medication someone else has prepared. This is a serious break in the control of medication because it prevents verifying the source of the drug, its cleanliness, or any of the eight "rights". Nurses who rely on this practice expose their patients to significant risk of harm and themselves to legal, regulatory, or disciplinary action.

Administering Without a Medication Administration Record (MAR)

Administering medication without the MAR is unsafe, as orders may have changed since you last looked at the MAR or you may miss a newly ordered medication. Having the MAR with you is also essential in order to perform the eight "rights" of medication administration. Finally, it is impossible to remember who refused, who was a no-show, and who received a PRN medication if you wait to document until after. If you chart before, you will make documentation errors because you can't know in advance which medications you will not give.

Administering Unidentified Medication

Inmates may have their own medications with them when they arrive at the facility, their family may bring in their medications, or the patient may have medication in their property that they were taking while at another correctional facility. While it may be tempting to use these, always positively identify what each of the medications are and that the label corresponds to the medication identity. Do not accept medications you cannot identify, are mixed in one container, or appear to be altered in any way.

Administering Someone Else's Medication to a Patient

Correctional nurses are always on the lookout for ways to deliver needed care in our resource-scarce environment. When a patient's medication is not available, sometimes nurses will take a dose from another patient's supply. Or nurses will hoard medications that should be returned to the pharmacy and use these to give other patients until the medication arrives or is found. Both practices are considered forms of drug diversion and are serious deviations from pharmacy law, which can expose the nurse to charges of wrongdoing. Borrowing medication is unnecessary when the following practices or arrangements are in place:

- A supply of stock medications is available to address unexpected needs, including antibiotics, insulin, antihypertensives, and inhalers.

- Newly arrived medication is put away for the patient as soon as it is received. Don't let medications that have been delivered from the pharmacy pile up in the warehouse or medication room.

- Medication carts or other storage are kept up-to-date with inmate movement and well organized so you can find a patient's medication easily.

- If you administer medication in the housing unit or in the yard, check before you leave your staging area for new orders or new admissions. Check also to see if there are medications that have been received but not yet put away.

- If the medication isn't listed on the MAR, check the orders because the prescription may have been discontinued or changed.

Additional information, including a list of medications that should not be crushed, may be found at correctionalnurse.net/quickstart.

Application Questions

The following application questions can help you learn about and apply the safety features involved in medication management at your facility.

1. List the specific ways that correctional officers at your facility contribute to medication safety.

2. What steps are taken at your facility when inmates are unruly in medication line?

3. How and when does the nurse perform hand hygiene during medication administration?

4. What are all the opportunities to transmit infection during medication administration, and what is in place to prevent transmission?

5. Are there risky medication administration practices at your facility? What can you do to reduce risk when you are administering medication?

6 Managing and Monitoring Treatment

Medication delivery is a complex process, and yet it is often thought of as just another task. In some correctional health care programs, specific individuals are given responsibility to "do meds" or are referred to as the "med nurse" – under the false assumption that all they do during the shift is pass out medication. Of course, medication delivery is just *one* aspect of the patient's treatment, and the nurse's responsibility to the patient is more than simply passing medication. It involves all aspects of the nursing process: assessment, diagnosis, outcomes identification, planning, and evaluating care. Additionally, the nurse retains responsibility for the process and outcomes of nursing care when medication delivery is delegated to a practical or vocational nurse or a certified medication aide. Responsibility also remains when correctional officers deliver medication at the facility. Nurses manage and monitor treatment by:

- Being accessible and alert to the patient or other's report of symptoms and side effects;

- Establishing good communication with the staff who are assigned to deliver medication;

- Being aware of the patient's living environment and factors that could affect their health condition and day-to-day experience;

- Advocating for the patient as necessary to ensure that nursing care and other ordered treatment is provided timely; and

- Taking steps to ensure safe delivery or administration of medications by licensed and unlicensed staff.

Med Line Tips

Medication line can be daunting for nurses new to the correctional setting. A nurse may be expected to administer medication to 200 or more inmates who gather in a line two, three, or four times a day. In addition, the nurse may run med line from a medication cart stationed near the dining hall or by the recreation yard or may need to roll the cart from housing unit to housing unit through all kinds of weather. Clearly this is different from how medication administration is done in other health care settings. Here are some tips to make running med line go more smoothly:

1. Make sure the medication cart or area is stocked with the things you are likely to need, including:

    - Patient medications;
    - MARs
    - Pen, highlighter, and notepad;
    - Forms (refusal, missing medication, error, sick call, etc.);
    - Current drug reference book;
    - Calculator;
    - Pill crusher and packets if needed;
    - Pill cups;
    - Water and drinking cups;
    - Waste receptacle; and

- Keys needed to access the medication room, cart, and narcotics container.

2. Take these steps before every med line:

   - Scan the MARs for any new medication orders or any new patients, and verify that each MAR indicates any allergies the patient may have.

   - Check to see that new medications are available to administer and, if not, where they are in the process of being dispensed and delivered.

   - Check for any medications that are expiring and need referral to a provider for renewal.

   - If you are unfamiliar with any medications, check a drug reference.

   - Make any calculations you need to administer the correct dose.

   - Perform hand hygiene.

3. When you are ready to administer medication, follow the same steps each time. This is called habituation and keeps you from skipping a step. Your consistency also makes it easier to manage inmate behavior when their cooperation is needed.

   - Ask security staff to assist in ensuring that the area is as quiet and free of distractions as possible.

   - Use two forms of identification to guarantee it is the right patient. Do not rely on your visual memory of what the patient looks like.

   - Locate the MAR corresponding to the patient's name and identification.

   - Scan the MAR for medications due.

   - Locate the medication and check the medication name, dose, time, and route against the MAR.

- Put the medication in a cup.

- Repeat for each medication that is due.

- State the name of each medication to the patient as you prepare to put it into the cup. If it is a new medication, confirm that the patient knows its purpose, major side effects, or precautions.

- Recheck the MAR and medications in the cup.

- Ask the patient if they have any questions about the medications.

- Watch the patient take the medication; watch for palming, and check the patient's oral cavity for cheeking. Beware of any distractions at this point because it may be an attempt at diversion.

- Have the patient put the medicine cup into the waste before leaving the medication cart or window.

- Document administration of each medication administered.

An audit tool to review nurse-administered medication practices can be found at correctionalnurse.net/quickstart. It is a good way to provide feedback to individual nurses regarding a process that often goes unnoticed until there is a significant problem with performance. It can also be used to spot system problems that nurses may need support to correct such as lack of custody support or inadequate equipment.

Addressing Side Effects, Questions, or Complaints

Expect to converse with patients when you administer or deliver medications. Many patients will have questions like "How long will it take before I feel better?" Often they will voice complaints like "This pill isn't working!" They may report side effects and refuse to take the medication. Nurses often initiate conversation with questions like "Do you know why you are taking this medication?" or "How are you feeling?" or "I am glad to see you take your medication today." These conversations are vital to treatment because they yield important information and help build rapport with the patient. But try to keep each conversation short so that other patients don't have to wait a long time and the med pass does not interrupt other scheduled activities or delay the escort officer from other duties. Also, do not escalate a patient's anger or distress. If a lengthy discussion is necessary, or the conversation is distracting or confrontational, ask the patient to wait until med line is over and then return to address the issue.

Medication treatment is an aspect of health care that receives a lot of complaints. There are many facets that can go awry such as the order not being transcribed, the medication was not delivered or mislaid, the side effects are intolerable, and so on. A nurse faces unhappy, disgruntled, or unwell inmates every day when administering medication, so it is worth the time to resolve issues before the problem grows.

Supporting Patients to Self-administer Medication

The nurse's role in self-medication programs emphasizes assessment, teaching, evaluation, and coaching patients to be responsible for their own health care.

Assessment

The first step is to evaluate whether the patient has the capacity or competence to care for themselves. This is an explicit competency of correctional nursing practice listed in the ANA's scope and standards of professional practice (2013). There are two reasons why we should assess competency: (1.) to ensure treatment is accomplished as prescribed; and (2.) to protect the patient from harm. Consider their answers to the following questions in determining whether a patient can administer their own medication.

- Does the patient want to administer their own medication?

- Is the patient able to tell the day and time accurately?

- Is the patient vulnerable to having the medication taken from them? This may be a characteristic of the patient (such as cognitive impairment) or the medication (one with high diversion value in the correctional setting).

- Is the patient able to follow instructions?

- Is the patient able to follow the rules of the self-administration program? For example, the steps to refill a medication or to obtain a renewal may be too complex for a particular patient.

- Is the dosing regimen simple enough for the patient to follow?

Patients with limited capacity may still be able to participate in self-administration if the program can be modified or adapted to the patient's strengths. The assessment will identify what aspects would best be modified if needed to support the patient's participation.

Patient Teaching

Each patient who is in a self-administration program needs to know about their medication(s) and how they are to be taken. Because low health literacy is a characteristic of many patients in the correctional setting, the nurse must take into account the patient's ability to understand the material when preparing and teaching patients about their medications. Information about how to assess health literacy and tools to work with patients who have low health literacy may be found at correctionalnurse.net/quickstart.

Here is a list of subjects that need to be covered when preparing patients for self-administration of medication.

- The medication's intended effect and dosing regimen (even if a patient has been on the medication before, this is a good time to check for and correct misunderstanding or misconceptions);

- The medication's side effects, including how to tolerate them and when to seek medical attention;

- The patient's allergy history and a discussion about how to differentiate side effects from an allergic reaction;

- Precautions the patient needs to be aware of and what action to take, including interactions with food, canteen products, or other medication, whether the medication will make the patient more sensitive to heat or light, dizziness upon standing, abrupt discontinuance of the drug, and so forth;

- The process or rules of the self-medication program and who to see or write to if they have problems or questions; and

- Any common concerns that are unique to practices at your facility.

Reviewing inmate grievances about medications is a good source of information about common concerns that might be addressed proactively during patient teaching.

Evaluation

Even with the best of intentions when learning something new or changing behavior, a person rarely gets it completely correct on their first try. Once the patient has been placed in a self-medication program, the nurse needs to follow up to see how the patient is doing, what questions they have, and what information needs to clarified or corrected. It is best to do this soon after the initial teaching (ideally by the end of the first week on the program) and then increase the time between evaluations thereafter. Have the patient bring the medication with them when they meet with you. Ask the patient how and when they are taking the medications, count the medication remaining, and determine if the remaining amount is correct. The nurse should also ask the patient if they have any questions, are experiencing side effects, or have any other problems. Advise the patient about how to manage side effects, answer questions, or take other action as needed to reduce barriers the patient is experiencing.

A nurse discovers a lot when following up in this way. For example, a patient who has taken only half the dose of prescribed antibiotics explained that he felt better so he decided to save the remainder for the next time. This is a great opportunity for the nurse to correct a misunderstanding about the treatment plan for his abscessed tooth. Besides correcting misunderstandings, it is also important to acknowledge and reinforce what the patient is doing well.

Coaching

Coaching differs from teaching in that it works with the patient's current knowledge and abilities to gain a new skill or improve performance. Coaching takes place in conjunction with an evaluation of the patient's adherence. If a patient, for example, forgets to take a daily dose because he sleeps in, he might do better if you suggest the dose be taken at another time of day or connect it to another activity that the patient does daily. Or, in another example, if the patient takes multiple medications and is confused about which one is taken when, you might develop a cheat sheet that the patient can use. The nurse can also use coaching to work with patients to prepare for their next provider appointment by suggesting subjects to bring up during the visit and information the provider will want to know about. The outcome of coaching about self-medication is better patient adherence with the plan of care, as well as the development of self-care skills that will benefit the patient when they return to the community. Information about how to identify patients likely to need coaching and strategies to support adherence can be found at correctionalnurse.net/quickstart.

Case Example – Self-administration

One day, a corrections officer delivered three grocery bags of medications to the medication room that were outdated and had been confiscated from inmates during a cell search of an entire housing unit. The manager includes this problem as a topic for the staff meeting the next day. Staff are asked to help develop as many solutions as possible to the problem of outdated medication being found in inmates' possession. What ideas will you suggest?

Specialized Medication Procedures

Most medications administered by nurses are oral or topical preparations. Medications that must be administered by other routes will most often take place in the clinic or inpatient setting. Insulin, tuberculin skin tests, and vaccination make up the majority of these. Supplies and equipment used in correctional facilities sometimes lag behind advances seen in hospitals and other health care settings. One of these is the continued use of multi-dose vials for multiple patients. Here is a list of tips to remember in using bulk stock multi-dose vials.

- Write the expiration date on a multi-use vial when it is first it is opened. These dates vary based upon the manufacturer, but to simplify this, some facilities opt for a general policy based upon the earliest expiration date (i.e. 28 days) unless otherwise specified.

- Cleanse multi-dose vials with 70% alcohol before inserting a needle into the vial.

- Never re-insert a used needle into a multi-use vial.

- Discard multi-dose vials if sterility is compromised.

Some injectable medications, inhalants, and other liquids may require refrigeration, so follow the pharmacy's direction for proper storage and maintenance of temperatures. There should be a refrigerator dedicated to medication storage, which is kept clean and free of food, laboratory specimens, and supplies. A thermometer should be kept in the refrigerator to verify that the temperature is maintained between 36°- 46° F. If temperatures are too high or low the pharmacy should be called for instructions. Temperatures in the refrigerator are read and recorded at least daily on a log.

Occasionally, specialized nursing procedures such as intravenous therapy, use of central IV lines, medication titration, methadone, and chemotherapy administration take place in correctional facilities. Because of the high level of skill required and infrequency of these procedures, correctional nurses may be intimidated. Regular skills fairs are one way to learn and keep skills in performing these less-frequent medication administration procedures up-to-date. Correctional nurses expect to continue developing their knowledge and skill, including the capacity to provide nursing care that hasn't been provided at the correctional facility before. Resources a nurse can access to learn a new procedure or skill include:

- Demonstrations by manufacturers or drug vendors;

- In-service and skills training provided by another correctional facility already providing the service;

- Continuing education offered by a local hospital or clinic;

- Courses or seminars provided by a local school of nursing;

Continuity of Care

One of the most important factors affecting inmates' willingness to follow the treatment plan is whether their symptoms are relieved and new ones not experienced. If patients don't feel better, they are not going to follow treatment recommendations. Increasing adherence to prescribed medication has been found to have a greater effect on health outcomes than any other specific form of medical treatment. Monitoring patients closely for symptom response, addressing side effects promptly, and eliminating barriers and other reasons for medication discontinuity increase the likelihood of treatment success with patients. These interventions are within correctional nurses' independent scope of practice and can therefore be implemented without specific provider orders.

Specific steps a nurse can take to support the patient's continuity of medication treatment are listed below.

1. Notify custody staff of patients whose medication requires:

    - Dietary restrictions or a special diet, for example, patients with diabetes or taking MAO inhibitors;

    - Work restrictions such as not driving or using machinery when a patient is taking medication that causes sedation;

    - Canteen (commissary) restrictions when, for example, a patient's salt intake or carbohydrates must be limited;

    - Housing restrictions, such as a lower bunk for a patient taking medication that causes dizziness or medically supervised housing for patients on medication that needs close monitoring (e.g. rehydration); and

- Environmental precautions, for example, limiting exposure for patient's taking heat or light sensitive medication.

2. Follow up appointments should be scheduled with appropriate health staff.

- *Nursing*: Schedule a nursing visit to check adherence by review of the MAR or the patient's own medication if on KOP; to collect serial data such as blood pressure, weight, blood glucose; and to find out from the patient if they are feeling better (intended effects) or experiencing side effects (unintended effects). Patients with poor adherence should be seen weekly, while those with better adherence can be seen monthly or quarterly.

- *Provider*: Appointments should be scheduled with the patient's provider(s) to review labs; to discuss progress, symptom relief, side effects, treatment adherence; and to adjust prescribed treatment as necessary. Provider appointments should be scheduled to coincide with the availability of lab or other monitoring measures (e.g. blood pressure, blood glucose). Appointments should also be scheduled so that the patient is seen when medication needs to be re-ordered.

- *Labs and Monitoring*: Schedule lab and other monitoring measures to coincide with provider appointments but take place in advance so that the data is available for review and discussion during the appointments. Be familiar with common lab work recommended for medications you are responsible for providing to patients, and help providers remember to order these when appropriate.

Case Example – Medication Adherence

Jessie has put in a sick call request because she is depressed and anxious. You see her later in the day; she is worried about her children, who are under the care of their aunt while Jessie is incarcerated. She is unable to sleep, tearful, and was sanctioned recently for not following orders. She is having difficulty getting along with her cellmate and prefers to stay in the corner of the dayroom. You note in her record that Jessie has diagnoses of schizoaffective disorder, asthma, and hypertension. She takes several different medications and misses taking them about half of the time. Jessie uses sick call frequently and has declared several medical emergencies for chest pain and shortness of breath, later diagnosed as anxiety. Jesse missed a recent mental health appointment and claimed she was not notified. She is unsure about her work and program assignments, and her appearance at the sick call is disheveled. What are the steps that can be taken to support this patient's adherence with prescribed medication?

Preventing and Addressing Unintended Effects

According to the World Health Organization (WHO), approximately 50% of patients with chronic illness do not take medications as prescribed; other studies have found compliance to be even less. This is also a problem in correctional settings. A verified, community-based dosage may be too high because the provider in the community was not aware that the patient was not taking the medication as prescribed. Now that the person is in custody, they develop symptoms of over-medication because their medication *is* being taken as prescribed. Jeff Keller, a well-known correctional physician calls this the "Compliance Trap" and advises that we all need to be wary of this potential risk.

Correctional nurses need to know the signs and symptoms of conditions that indicate an unintended side effect or adverse reaction to medication, especially those common to patients being treated in correctional settings. When these symptoms develop, the nurse is most likely to see the patient first, identify the problem, initiate prompt treatment, and follow up with the patient. Common effects and reactions are listed below.

- *Allergic reaction or anaphylaxis*: Drugs most often associated with allergic reactions include anticonvulsants, insulin (animal sourced), penicillin and related antibiotics, sulfa drugs, vaccines, and iodine-based x-ray contrast dyes. Anaphylaxis is a medical emergency, and the facility should have a written protocol that is used to initiate treatment.

- *Heat exhaustion and heat stroke*: Environmental conditions and institution rules can put inmates at risk of heat exhaustion and stroke because individuals can not regulate the temperature in their cell, or may be required to work outside when the temperature is high, or may have limited access to water. Individuals taking psychotropic medication, diuretics, antiparkinsonian or anticholinergic medication, amphetamines, and beta blockers are particularly at risk. Correctional facilities typically have an established policy and practice to prevent heat exhaustion and stroke. See correctionalnurse.net/quickstart for a comprehensive report on the problem of heat in correctional settings, which includes the policies and procedures of state and federal correctional facilities beginning on page 91. If your facility does not have one, use this resource and/or contact other correctional facilities and ask for a copy to adapt to your site.

- *Photosensitivity*: Similar to heat exhaustion, inmates often cannot control their exposure to light and, if taking certain medications, may experience extreme sunburn or urticarial reactions. A list of these medications and tips on prevention and treatment is provided in an article published by the Institute for Safe Medication Practices (IMSP) that can be found at correctionalnurse.net/quickstart.

- *Hyponatremia*: This is a condition identified by low sodium levels and can be caused by several triggers, including certain medications (e.g. SSRIs, haloperidol, MAO inhibitors, diuretics, some chemotherapeutic agents, chlorpropamide, and use of IVs). Treatment will depend on the likely cause and may include water restriction, electrolyte monitoring, and vital sign monitoring.

- *Complications from psychotropic medication:* Extrapyramidal symptoms, tardive dyskinesia, serotonin syndrome, lithium toxicity, neuroleptic malignant syndrome, and metabolic syndrome are each complications of treatment with psychotropic medications. Unless you were a psychiatric nurse before transferring to corrections, you are probably not familiar with any of these. Because more than one half the population in correctional settings have mental health problems, *all* correctional nurses must be familiar with the assessment and treatment of psychiatric disorders, including the medications, the side effects, and adverse reactions. Contact the facility psychiatrist, nurse practitioner, or physician's assistant for their help to increase your knowledge in this area, especially if mental health nursing is new to you.

Application Questions

The following questions are designed to help you find out about how treatment is managed and monitored at your facility.

1. Compare medication administration to the list of med line tips. Are there any missing supplies, equipment, or steps that you might want to put in place?

2. What practices do you use to ensure that you are administering the right medication to the right patient?

3. How would you evaluate a patient's readiness to take their own medications, if self-administration is allowed at your facility?

4. Compare the safety points for use of multi-use vials to the practices at your facility. Are there any improvements that could be made?

5. How is patient adherence to medication monitored at your facility? What steps are taken to support patient adherence?

6. How is medication continuity ensured at your facility?

7 Timeliness of Medication Treatment

Timeliness of medication treatment is one of the most vexing challenges in correctional settings. This is because there are so many other things that compete for the same time and so many steps to ensure that prescription orders are carried out. Being aware of standards for timeliness of medication treatment and creative in developing solutions to challenges inherent in the correctional settings distinguish successful correctional nurses. The following are some tips to meet timeliness requirements.

Standards for Timeliness

Now that we have described all the steps involved in getting medication to patients in a correctional facility, let's consider parameters for timeliness in implementing prescribed treatment. A patient being treated for third degree burns should receive as-needed pain medication within minutes of asking; a patient with pneumonia needs to take antibiotics as often as prescribed; and a diabetic patient should eat shortly after taking insulin. Meeting these needs for timeliness can be tricky in correctional facilities.

Time from the Order to First Dose

There should be a standard time frame for how long a medication should take to arrive after an order is sent to the pharmacy. Each order must be monitored or tracked so that, when a deviation occurs, it is identified and addressed quickly. If the order is written as STAT or immediate, the patient should receive medication from emergency stock or the pharmacy before leaving the clinic. These orders are the exception in correctional settings; the majority are written to start when the medication has arrived. Some facilities may administer from bulk stock until the patient-specific prescription arrives. When the standard time frame is only a day or two, administering from bulk stock is not necessary unless the provider indicates that initiating treatment is urgent. Unacceptable delays in treatment can occur when orders are not sent to the pharmacy promptly or the medication is not unpacked and put away promptly when it is received from the pharmacy. It may be necessary for additional staff to step in and help or for the staffing plan to be adjusted to meet the expected time frames.

Refills

Typically, the pharmacy dispenses only a portion of the total quantity of medication that was ordered, and it will be necessary to request periodic refills until the order runs out. For example, medication orders for patients with chronic diseases are typically written for 90 – 180 days, but most correctional pharmacies only dispense a 30-day supply. The nurse or the patient, if it is a self-administered medication, will need to request a refill. The refill needs to be requested early enough that the medication will be dispensed and arrive before the last dose is taken. Usually there is some visual indicator on the package that shows when the refill should be requested; in most cases, this is 7-10 days before the last dose.

It is common for patients who self-administer medication to forget to ask for a refill in time. If it is a critical medication, the patient will then have to be treated from bulk stock. On the flip side, other patients request refills so early that the pharmacy cannot dispense. Missed doses and disgruntled patients can be prevented with patient education and coaching. For nurse-administered medication, note those that need refilling in preparation for or immediately after each med line. Check the refill numbers or time frame of the order to know if there are no more refills and a renewal is necessary instead. Some pharmacies provide a sticky label that can be peeled off, put on a sheet of paper, and sent to the pharmacy to request refills. This saves time and the potential for transcription error.

Renewals

Every prescription has an end date; when this date approaches, the provider should re-evaluate the patient's condition. The provider may renew the order, write a new order, or let the order expire. In order to ensure treatment continuity, the patient needs to see the provider, the orders need to be written, and the medication must be dispensed and received at the facility before the existing order runs out. This takes coordination and cooperation. One way to ensure that treatment continues is, *at the time the initial order is written,* schedule the patient for a provider visit to coincide with the prescription end date. Another is for the pharmacy to send a list of patients whose medication orders are expiring in the next 30 days; the nurse can use the list to schedule appointments. Yet another is for the pharmacy to notify the provider in advance of orders that are expiring. Some systems rely on the patient to request a provider appointment, but because the patient has no way of knowing the provider's schedule, they are inevitably seen late and either miss doses or an urgent order is written without the patient being seen. As part of the daily preparation for medication administration or the review of new MARs, nurses should make note of those patients whose orders are running out and follow up to ensure that they see a provider.

Dosing Schedules

The time, methods, and location for medication delivery are a joint decision of the facility administrator and the health care leadership. The primary objective is to administer medication in a manner that is timely, safe, and optimally therapeutic. Typically, facilities will have one or two scheduled times when most medications are administered. While medication can be administered at other times of the day based upon the prescriber's order, all once-daily doses usually are given at either the morning or evening pill line. Medication lines should be timed to correspond with the intended purpose of the drug. As an example, medications with sedative effects should be given at bedtime, not early evening or during the day, if at all possible.

Sometimes a provider will order medication to be administered at times when health care staff are not on duty. For example, a patient with HS medications should not be housed in an area that is only staffed on day shift unless special accommodations are made. These could include allowing the patient to self-administer, flexing the schedule of one of the nursing staff, seeing if the prescriber would consider dosing at a time other than at night, or moving the patient to an area that is staffed to administer HS meds. Less adequate solutions are to prepare and package a single dose and give it to the patient or to custody to give to the patient at night. This has the same disadvantages of pre-pouring described earlier; in addition, the patient may not take it correctly, and it inappropriately relies on custody to perform a task for which they are neither trained nor credentialed.

Daily Delivery

Timely administration of medication is a particular challenge for correctional nurses. Many correctional facilities have established a 1-hour window before or after the designated time for medication to be administered. If you struggle with timeliness of medication administration, you may want to consider using the approach recommended by the Institute for Safe Medication Practices (ISMP), which is summarized here.

- Identify the medications used at your facility that are time-critical or should be administered *within 30 minutes* of the scheduled time. The ISMP has identified the following as time-critical medications:

88

Table 7.1. Time-Critical Medications
Antibiotics
Anticoagulants
Insulin
Anticonvulsants
Immunosuppressive agents
Medication that must be administered within a specific time period
Medications that must be administered apart from other medications for optimal therapeutic effect
Pain medication
Medications prescribed to be taken every four hours or more frequently
Medications that must be administered in relation to meals (before, after or with)

- Develop a method to administer time-critical medications within the window. One solution is to admit these patients to an inpatient unit or house them on one or two living units designated for inmates on time-critical medication. Another option is to establish a time-critical medication line that differs from the time for administration of medications that are not time critical.

- The number of patients on time-critical medications should be small, given that these are correctional settings and not acute care facilities. If there are a lot of QID orders or other medications that are identified as time-critical, nursing must collaborate with the facility medical director to develop alternatives for appropriate treatment of these patients.

- Daily, weekly, or monthly doses *do not have a timeliness window* if given on the day it is due. It has long been recommended that the dose be timed to some other event (e.g. after breakfast or the morning med line) to help the patient remember. These patients could be scheduled on a separate med line so that they do not slow down med line for other patients or scheduled among all the med lines. Weekly or monthly doses could be scheduled as clinic appointments rather than on med line.

- Medications administered more frequently than daily (e.g. BID, TID, QID) should be given within the window of *an hour* before or after the scheduled time.

The majority of patients on medication in a correctional setting should be on daily dosing schedules. It is worth looking at patients on multiple daily doses and asking prescribers to consider less frequent schedules. Often prescribers are unaware of the challenges nurses have with timely medication administration and are willing to alter orders. Patients also complain about long waits in med line and may be more willing to adhere to less frequent dosages.

Sometimes nurses are pressured to abandon one or more of the "rights" of medication administration (right patient, right medication, right dose, etc.) in the interest of speed because there are too many inmates to medicate in the time available. Here are some options, in addition to those discussed above, to manage this problem without abandoning your safety practices.

- Suggest establishing a self-administration program if one does not exist.

- Deliver self-administered medication in another line.

- Suggest using the commissary or some other way to provide over-the-counter medications rather than med line.

PRN or "As-needed" Medications

A nurse should assess the patient's condition shortly after the patient has requested a PRN, administer the medication based upon the nursing assessment, and document the findings and intervention in the health record. It is difficult to administer as-needed prescriptions correctly in correctional settings. Because inmate access to a nurse is limited by custody schedules, meal times, lock-down time, and visiting, neither the request for a PRN nor the nursing response can be guaranteed timely. Remedies to this problem are to allow the patient to self-administer the medication or admit the patient to an inpatient or other unit where nursing staff are readily available to administer PRN medication when it is needed.

Court Appearances

Many inmates are held in county jails, juvenile detention facilities, or prison reception areas while going through a court proceeding that can last anywhere from just a day or two to several years. Whenever an inmate goes to court, arrangements must be made to continue medical care, even if the court is only two blocks away. Usually the facility has a way to notify the health care program of those going to court on a given day; this information is typically available the night before the inmate goes to the transport area or court holding area. A nurse receiving this notification should review the MAR and the health record to determine what arrangements need to be made to continue treatment while at court. Some correctional systems allow inmates to carry their medications to be taken during the day, while others set up a time for the nurse to go administer the medications. Sometimes the medication is given before they leave (i.e. once daily medications or perhaps just the morning dose).

Riots, Lockdowns and other Facility Emergencies

Consider this situation: just as you are preparing for morning med pass, a man-down alarm is sounded. Your partner is assigned to emergencies today, so he grabs the emergency bag and heads to the announced floor. A few minutes later, as you are rolling the cart out of the medication room, a call comes in. The man-down is an officer assault, so the entire facility is in lockdown, and morning medication rounds are cancelled. Now what?

This is when that good working relationship you have built with custody staff and the respect you have demonstrated for security practices really comes into play! Even though security is a priority in a correctional facility, as a nurse, you still have an obligation to make sure that needed medical care – including medication – is provided in a timely manner. By having a good working relationship and mutual understanding of the need for timely administration of medication, often a solution can be reached about how medication will be delivered when med pass has been cancelled or delayed. Alternate methods for delivery of time-critical medications, which may include cell-side administration or escort of patients to the clinic or another area to receive needed medication, will all be much better facilitated if you have "earned" the cooperation of your custody colleagues.

It can be hard to negotiate a satisfactory solution in a crisis when staff are agitated, anxious, or angry. It is, therefore, a best practice to have a policy or procedure established jointly by custody and health care *in advance of a crisis* that describes what to do when medication delivery is cancelled or delayed. The following are the steps that should be taken by nurses when medication administration is cancelled or delayed.

- Notify your chain of command of the cancellation or delay.

- Review all medications to identify those that are time-critical.

- Confer with custody about how time-critical medications will be administered.

- Shift medications that are not time-critical to another medication time.

- Consult with a provider about those patients where it is not clear whether the medication is time-critical or not.

Multiple episodes of cancellation or delay should be addressed right away as a quality improvement project; protocols for prolonged cancellation such as a lockdown should be part of the correctional facility's incident response plan. If delays and cancellations are a frequent occurrence, it may be worthwhile to mark the blister card or medication package in some way to denote time-critical medications and/or maintain a roster or alert system that identifies inmates who are on time-critical medications.

Case Example

A patient is getting ready for an offsite specialty procedure the next day and has a medication that he is to receive at 5:00 pm today. As you are taking it to the housing unit, you are informed that the unit is in lockdown because of a disturbance. The officers will not let you into the unit to administer the medication. If the patient does not receive the medication soon, the appointment will have to be cancelled. What actions are available to you so that the patient receives their medication timely?

Application Questions

Here are some questions to get you thinking about challenges and solutions to medication timeliness at your facility.

1. Are medications administered so that the time interval between doses is neither too long nor too short?

2. What are five medications that are time-sensitive for medication administration?

3. How long, on average, does it take for the first dose of medication to be administered after an order is written?

4. How long, on average, does it take to get refills delivered at your facility? How long do renewals typically take?

5. What measures does your facility have to ensure that inmates receive medications as ordered when they go out to court?

6. What is the procedure you follow if a facility disturbance or emergency prevents you from administering medication?

Conclusion

Correctional nurses have expanded roles in managing medications in the correctional setting because they are often only one of a few health care professionals onsite. Nurses new to correctional health care are often overwhelmed at the scope of responsibility they have for the health and well-being of their patients, particularly medication management.

Correctional nursing practice conforms to state regulation, laws, and rules, as well as to standards of practice to ensure that services are consistent with community expectations. Correctional nurses are familiar with the terminology used to communicate about medications and the references or resources that are used to assist in medication management. They are responsible for obtaining medication from a pharmacy and making sure that medications are stored correctly, kept under proper control, and each dose accounted for.

Custody staff and the command staff at correctional facilities provide access to patients and security during medication administration. Nurses must comply with security requirements and develop a collaborative relationship with these professionals so that security is maintained while at the same time ensuring that treatment is provided as ordered.

Maintaining order and managing inmate behavior while administering medication is critical to maintaining a nurse's personal safety. The inmate population and the correctional setting offer ample room for medication error. Adhering to the eight "rights" of medication administration is an essential part of nursing practice in reducing the likelihood of error.

Incarceration provides opportunity for nurses to make a significant impact on the health and well-being of patients. Teaching and coaching about the role of medication in treating disease or injury may last throughout a patient's lifetime. Helping patients to achieve symptom improvement and preventing side effects is the most significant contribution a nurse can make in medication management.

After all is said and done, here is the sound advice about medication administration that we heard from one of the experienced correctional nurses we interviewed while working on this *Quick Start* book:

1. Know and double-check allergies.

2. Follow the eight "rights."

3. Pay attention to refusals – get the "what" and "why". Ask the patient.

4. Make sure patients take the medications. Check the mouth, and be astute.

5. Be vigilant to prevent diversion and misuse.

Ann Cline, RN BSN, Multnomah County Health Department, Corrections Health Division, June 17, 2015.

References and Resources

The following sources were consulted for fact accuracy in this book. Citation within the text was avoided to improve readability. Learn more about many of the topics in this book by obtaining these documents or online sources. Find other Quick Start resources at correctionalnurse.net/quickstart.

American Correctional Association. (2002). *Performance Based Standards for Correctional Health Care*. Retrieved August 19, 2015 from http://www.aca.org/standards/healthcare/

American Nurses Association. (2013). *Correctional Nursing: Scope and Standards of Practice.* Silver Springs, MD: American Nurses Association.

Bicknell, M., Brew, I., Cooke, C., Duncall, H., Palmer, J., & Robinson, J. (2011). *Safer Prescribing in Prisons: Guidance for Clinicians*. Royal College of General Practitioners, Secure Environments Group. Retrieved January 15, 2016 from http://www.rpharms.com/news-story-downloads/prescribinginprison.pdf.

Brown, M.T. & Bussell, J.K. (2011). Medication adherence: WHO cares? *Mayo Clinic Proceedings*, 86(4): 304-314.

Bonsall, L.M. (2011). 8 rights of medication administration. Retrieved June 17, 2016, from http://www.nursingcenter.com/ncblog/may-2011/8-rights-of-medication-administration

Burrow, G.F., Knox, C.M., & Villanueva, H. (2006). Nursing in the primary care setting. In M. Puisis (ed.) *Clinical Practice in Correctional Medicine*, Second Edition, pp. 426-459. Philadelphia, PA: Elsevier Inc.

Centers for Disease Control and Prevention. (2014). *Prescription Drug Overdose in the United States: Fact Sheet*. Retrieved September 30, 2015, from http://www.cdc.gov/homeandrecreationalsafety/overdose/facts.html.

Dart, R.C., Borron, S.W., Caravati, E. M., et.al. (2009). Expert consensus guidelines for stocking of antidotes in hospitals that provide emergency care. *Annals of Emergency Medicine*, 54(3): 386-394.

Ehret, M.J., Barta, W., Maruca, A., et al. (2013). Medication adherence among female inmates with bipolar disorder: Results from a randomized controlled trail. *Psychological Services*, 10(1): 106-114.

Gettig, J.P. (2007). Drug information availability and preferences of health care professionals in Illinois: A pilot survey study. *Drug Information Journal*, 42: 263-272.

Grissinger, M. (2010). Tablet splitting-Only if you "half" to. *Pharmacy & Therapeutics* 35(2): 69-70.

Grohs, M. (March-April 2015). Dispensing medications. Retrieved January 20, 2016, from www.correctionsforum.net

Harmon, R.E. (2013). Mental health. In Schoenly, L. & Knox, C.M. (ed.) *Essentials of Correctional Nursing*, pp. 221-245. New York, NY: Springer Publishing Company LLC.

Holt, D.W.E. (2015). *Heat in US Prisons and Jails: Corrections and the Challenge of Climate Change*. Sabin Center for Climate Change Law, Columbia Law School. Retrieved February 21, 2016, from http://nicic.gov/library/031204

Institute for Safe Medication Practices. (2011). *Acute Care Guidelines for Timely Administration of Scheduled Medications.* Retrieved February 12, 2016, from http://www.ismp.org/tools/guidelines/acutecare/tasm.pdf

James, D.J. & Glaze, L.E. (2006). *Mental Health Problems of Prison and Jail Inmates.* U.S. Department of Justice, Officer of Justice Programs, Bureau of Justice Statistics. Retrieved June 16, 2015, from http://www.bjs.gov/content/pub/pdf/mhppji.pdf

Knox, C.M. (June 21, 2013). *Drug diversion or bad habits?* Retrieved January 20, 2016, from http://essentialsofcorrectionalnursing.com/2013/06/21/drug-diversion-or-bad-habits/

Knox, C.M. (June 26, 2014). *Identifying prescription drug misuse and abuse.* Retrieved January 20, 2016, from http://essentialsofcorrectionalnursing.com/2014/06/26/identifying-prescription-drug-misuse-and-abuse/

Knox, C. M. (July 3, 2014). *Preventing diversion of prescription drugs in prison and jail.* Retrieved January 20, 2016, from http://essentialsofcorrectionalnursing.com/2014/07/03/preventing-diversion-of-prescription-drugs-in-prison-and-jail/

Knox, C.M. (June 17, 2015). *Six challenges managing medications that make correctional nursing unique.* Retrieved February 22, 2016, from http://essentialsofcorrectionalnursing.com/2015/06/17/six-challenges-managing-medications-that-make-correctional-nursing-unique/

Knox, C.M. (August 28, 2015). *Communication and medication management.* Retrieved September 30, 2015, from http://essentialsofcorrectionalnursing.com/2015/08/28/communication-and-medication-management/

Knox, C. M. (September 4, 2015). *Knowledge resources for medication management*. Retrieved September 30, 2015, from http://essentialsofcorrectionalnursing.com/2015/09/04/knowle dge-resources-for-medication-management/

Kripalani S, Yao X, & Haynes B. (2007). Interventions to enhance medication adherence in chronic medical conditions. *Archives of Internal Medicine*, 167(6): 540-549.

LaFerney, M.C. (2010). Dealing with drug diversion. *Reflections on Nursing Leadership*. 36(2).

Maruschak, L. M., Berzofsky, M., & Unangst J. (2015) *Medical Problems of State and Federal Prisoners and Jail Inmates, 2011-12*. U.S. Department of Justice, Officer of Justice Programs, Bureau of Justice Statistics. Accessed June 16, 2015, from http://www.bjs.gov/content/pub/pdf/mpsfpji1112.pdf

McClure, S.R., O'Neal, B.C., Grauer, D., & Couldry, R.J. (2011). Compliance with recommendations for prevention and detection of controlled-substance diversion in hospitals. *American Journal of Health-System Pharmacy*. 68: 689-694

Mills, A., Lathlean, J., Forrester, A., Van Veenhuyzen, W. & Gray, R. (2011). Prisoners' experiences of antipsychotic medication: Influences on adherence. *The Journal of Forensic Psychiatry & Psychology*, 22(1): 110-125.

Mitchell, J. (January 2014). *Oral Dosage Forms That Should Not Be Crushed*. Institute for Safe Medication Practices.

Mooney, D.H. (2013). Investigating and make a case for drug diversion. *Journal of Nursing Regulation,* 4(1): 9-13.

National Commission on Correctional Health Care. (2014). *Standards for Health Services in Jails*. Chicago, IL: National Commission on Correctional Health Care.

National Commission on Correctional Health Care. (2014). *Standards for Health Services in Prisons*. Chicago, IL: National Commission on Correctional Health Care.

National Coordinating Council for Medication Error Reporting and Prevention (NCCMERP). (June 30, 2015). *About Medication Errors. What is a Medication Error?* Retrieved February 7, 2016, from http://www.nccmerp.org/about-medication-errors

National Coordinating Council for Medication Error Reporting and Prevention (NCCMERP). (June 2, 2005). *At Risk Behaviors by Healthcare Professionals Associated with Medication Errors*. Retrieved June 15, 2015, from http://www.nccmerp.org/council/council999-06-29.html

Ndosi, M. & Newell, R. (2010). Medicine information sources used by nurses at the point of care. *Journal of Clinical Nursing,* 19: 2659-2661.

O luga, A. & McGuire, M.J. (2014). Adherence and health costs. *Risk Management Health Policy,* 7: 35-44. Retrieved January 24, 2016, from http://www.ncbi.nlm.nih.gov/pmc/articles/PMC3934668/

Phillips, A. (2014). Prescribing in prison: Complexities and considerations. *Nursing Standard,* 28(21): 46-50.

Phillips, D. (2012). Wellbutrin®: Misuse and abuse by incarcerated individuals. *Journal of Addiction Nursing,* 23: 65-69.

Sabaté, E., ed. (2003). *Adherence to Long Term Therapies: Evidence for Action*. Geneva, Switzerland: World Health Organization. Retrieved January 24, 2015, from http://www.who.int/chp/knowledge/publications/adherence_report/en/

Schoenly, L. (August 28, 2015). *Crushing injury: Are you helping or harming when you crush pills?* Retrieved September 30, 2015, from http://correctionalnurse.net/?s=crushing+medications

Schoenly, L. (August 25, 2015). *Time crunch: What to do when med pass is cancelled.* Retrieved September 30, 2015, from http://correctionalnurse.net/time-crunch-what-to-do-when-med-pass-is-cancelled/

Schoenly, L. (August 5, 2014). *Legal history of correctional nursing, Part 1.* Retrieved September 30, 2015, from http://correctionalnurse.net/?s=legal+history+of+correctional+nursing.

Schoenly, L. (2013). Safety for the nurse and patient. In L. Schoenly & C. Knox, (Ed.) *Essentials of Correctional Nursing.* New York, NY: Springer Publishing Company, 73-74.

Schoenly, L. (2012). *DOTs and dashes: Direct observation therapy pointers for correctional nurses.* Retrieved September 15, 2015, from http://correctionalnurse.net/dots-and-dashes-direct-observation-therapy-pointers-for-correctional-nurses/

Schoenly, L. (2012). *Risky business: Pre-pour meds in jails and prisons.* Retrieved September 15, 2015, from http://correctionalnurse.net/risky-business-pre-pour-meds-in-jails-and-prisons/

Schoenly, L. (n.d.). *Four ways your patient can help you avoid a medication error.* Retrieved September 15, 2015, from http://correctionalnurse.net/four-ways-your-patient-can-help-you-avoid-a-medication-error/

Schoenly, L. (n.d.). *A pre-flight checklist before rolling out of the med room.* Retrieved January 20, 2016, from http://correctionalnurse.net/a-pre-flight-checklist-before-rolling-out-of-the-med-room/

Schoenly, L. (n.d.). *8 medication rights-not 5.* Retrieved January 20, 2016, from http://correctionalnurse.net/8-medication-rights-not-5/

Schoenly, L. (n.d.). *Verbal order safety tips.* Retrieved January 20, 2016, from http://correctionalnurse.net/verbal-order-safety-tips/

Schoenly, L. (n.d.). *Patient identification: Is the right patient getting that medication?* January 20, 2016, from http://correctionalnurse.net/patient-identification-it-the-right-patient-getting-that-medication/

Schoenly, L. (n.d.). *Are you a borrower or a hoarder?* Retrieved January 20, 2016, from http://correctionalnurse.net/are-you-a-borrower-or-a-hoarder/

Schoenly, L (n.d.). *Making ends meet: The blunt end and sharp end of clinical error.* Retrieved January 20, 2016, from http://correctionalnurse.net/making-ends-meet-the-blunt-end-and-sharp-end-of-clinical-error/

Schoenly, L. (n.d.). *Multi-dose vials: Risk and reality in corrections.* Retrieved January 20, 2016, from http://correctionalnurse.net/multi-dose-vials-risk-and-reality-in-corrections/

Schoenly, L. (n.d.). *Are you imprisoned by a messy med room?* Retrieved June 15, 2015, from http://correctionalnurse.net/are-you-imprisoned-by-a-messy-med-room/

Schoenly, L. (n.d.). *Personal safety during medication administration.* Retrieved June 15, 2015, from http://correctionalnurse.net/personal-safety-during-medication-administration/

The National Center on Addiction and Substance Abuse at Columbia University. (2010). *Behind bars II: Substance abuse and America's prison population.* New York, NY: The National Center on Addiction and Substance Abuse at Columbia University. Retrieved from http://www.casacolumbia.org/addiction-research/reports/substance-abuse-prison-system-2010.

U.S. Department of Justice, Office of Diversion Control. (2013). *Code of Federal Regulations 21 Part 1300*. Retrieved May 30, 2015, from http://www.deadiversion.usdoj.gov/21cfr/cfr/2100cfrt.htm.

Velligan, D.I., Weiden, P.J., Sajatovic, M. et al. (2010). Assessment of adherence problems in patients with serious and persistent mental illness: recommendations from the Expert Consensus Guidelines. *Journal of Psychiatric Practice*, 16(1): 34-45.

Velligan, D.I., Weiden, P.J., Sajatovic, M. et al. (2010). Strategies for addressing adherence problems in patients with serious and persistent mental illness: Recommendations from the Expert Consensus Guidelines. *Journal of Psychiatric Practice*, 16(5): 306-324.

Vera, M. (2012). *List of Common Drugs & Their Antidotes That Nurses Should Know!* Retrieved September 15, 2015, from http://nurseslabs.com/list-of-common-drugs-their-antidotes-that-nurses-should-know/

Vrabel, R. (2010). Identifying and dealing with drug diversion. *Health Management Technology*, 31(12): 1-5.

About the Authors

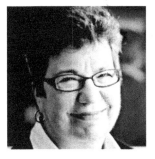

Catherine M. Knox MN, RN, CCHP-RN has more than three decades of leadership experience in correctional health care. Catherine has consulted since 2001 and in this capacity has managed the start- up and initial operation of contract health care programs, provided expert consultation to other correctional systems, and monitored delivery of correctional health care on behalf of the court.

She is a recipient of the "Distinguished Service Award" from the American Correctional Health Services Association (ACHSA) and the "Bernard Harrison Award of Merit" from the NCCHC.

Catherine co-authored the *Essentials of Correctional Nursing* with Lorry Schoenly published by Springer in 2013. She helped write a white paper on *Nurses Scope of Practice and Delegation Authority* published in 2014 by the NCCHC. More recently she contributed a chapter about medication adherence to the *Oxford Textbook on Correctional Psychiatry* published by the Oxford University Press in 2015. Look for an upcoming publication by Catherine on Work Environments that Support Correctional Nursing Practice in *Correctional Health Care – Practice, Administration and Law* to be published by Civic Research Institute in 2016.

Catherine splits her time between homes in Sedona, Arizona and Portland, Oregon enjoying the best of both climates. Her interests include travel, photography, and hiking.

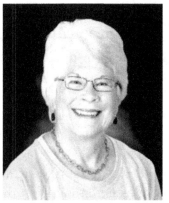**Gayle F. Burrow MPH, BSN, CCHP-RN** is a correctional health care consultant with experience that spans over thirty years. Her practice has been in a large urban jail system which included nursing care, leadership and management. Gayle is a recipient of the "Distinguished Service Award" from the American Correctional Health Services Association (ACHSA) and the "Public Health Leadership Award" from the Multnomah County Health Department.

Gayle has expanded into consulting on corrections health issues, a lead surveyor for NCCHC, participating in the blogging team for the Essentials of Correctional Nursing website, and board positions with corrections health membership organizations. Gayle previously wrote about the role of correctional nurses in delivery of primary care in the *Clinical Practice of Correctional Medicine* (2006).

Her home focus is keeping track of four grandchildren and maintaining a yard and garden in Portland, Oregon which is certified as a wildlife habitat.

About the Series Editor

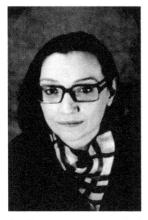 **Lorry Schoenly, PhD, RN, CCHP-RN**, is a nurse author and educator specializing in the field of correctional health care. She provides consulting services to jails and prisons across the country on projects to improve professional nursing practice and patient safety. She began her corrections experience in the New Jersey Prison System where she created and implemented education for nurses, physicians, dentists, and site managers. Before "accidentally" finding correctional healthcare, she practiced in critical care and orthopaedic specialties.

Dr. Schoenly actively promotes correctional nursing through social media outlets and increases the visibility of the specialty through her popular blog – correctionalnurse.net. Her podcast, Correctional Nursing Today, reviews correctional healthcare news and interviews correctional health care leaders. She is the recipient of the "B. Jaye Anno Award of Excellence in Communication" from the National Commission on Correctional Health Care.

For the past seven years, Dr. Schoenly has helped other nurses become nurse educators as a visiting professor in the graduate program of Chamberlain College of Nursing where she teaches in the nurse educator track.

When not writing, speaking, and consulting on correctional nursing practice, Lorry can be found reading Jane Austen, exploring civil war battlefields, or building Lego towers with her kindergartner grandson. She resides in the mountains of northcentral Pennsylvania.

66587927R00066